BARBARA McCOOL
Department of Health Administration
School of Nursing
Duke University

MONTAGUE BROWN
Department of Health Administration
Duke University

THE MANAGEMENT RESPONSE:

Conceptual, Technical and Human Skills of Health Administration

SAUNDERS SERIES IN
HEALTH CARE ORGANIZATION
AND ADMINISTRATION

1977

W. B. SAUNDERS COMPANY

PHILADELPHIA • LONDON • TORONTO

W. B. Saunders Company: West Washington Square
Philadelphia, PA   19105

1 St. Anne's Road
Eastbourne, East Sussex BN21 3UN, England

1 Goldthorne Avenue
Toronto, Ontario M8Z 5T9, Canada

Library of Congress Cataloging in Publication Data

McCool, Barbara.

The management response.

(Saunders series in health care organization and administration)

1. Health services administration.   I. Brown, Montague,
  joint author.   II. Title.   III. Series.

RA393.M23   658'.91'3621   76–41534

ISBN 0–7216–5891–1

The Management Response   ISBN   0-7216-5891-1

Last digit is the print number: 9   8   7   6   5   4   3   2   1

To Bill, Mary, Barney, and Minnie

FOREWORD

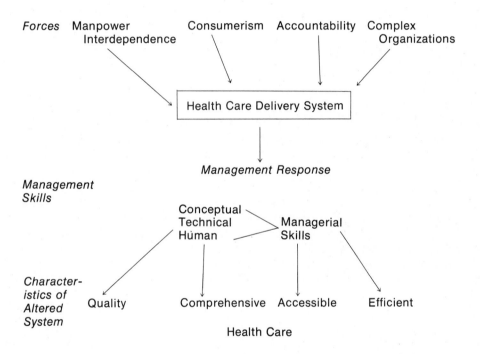

Forces Manpower   Consumerism Accountability Complex
            Interdependence   Organizations

Health Care Delivery System

Management Response

Management
Skills

Conceptual
Technical   Managerial
Human   Skills

Character-
istics of
Altered   Quality   Comprehensive Accessible   Efficient
System

Health Care

   This book is intended to develop the conceptual, technical, and human skills of managers.

   Each learning unit is organized around the model presented above. Attention is paid to the impact of environmental forces (internal and external) that shape the manager's perception of needed action and change. Each learning module is written to stand alone, although each also draws from and extends some of the thinking developed in earlier chapters. The objective of each learning module is spelled out at the beginning of the module, and examples, exercises, and questions are offered to assist the reader in grasping the concepts presented. We believe that a critical distinction that separates the effective manager from the mediocre manager is the ability to *think* about situations and form mental pictures of possible consequences of action to test out the appropriateness of any given solution. The systems analyst and the operations researcher carry this process to large-scale mathematical models and run computer analyses of alternatives. Those less mathematically oriented develop descriptive and written models. Some spend four to six years studying management theory and techniques in order to relate in the complex organizations of today's world. This book attempts to bring some of the less quantitative conceptual models to those who will not go through such extensive training but who expend their energy primarily upon the management skills and services that support the medical effort.

Each of the chapters deals with a conceptual, technical, or human management area in a way that will enhance the manager's skill in *thinking* about the management task. It is hoped that these presentations will improve the management capability of department heads, supervisors, and others who must delegate authority.

Thus, the audience for this book is the department head, supervisor, head nurse, team leader, and those trained primarily in management but who need a review. These are individuals who must increasingly demonstrate the leadership and enlightened conduct that typically emerge from continuing education in the area of management knowledge and skills. This training should equip them to cope more intelligently with interrelated departments and demands being made by the forces that are influencing and changing the health care system and the demands imposed upon it. This middle management group needs specific conceptual, human, and technical skills in order to perform its job effectively. The acquisition of these skills and how they will affect the future delivery of health care is the subject of this book.

CONTENTS

Unit I

CONCEPTUAL SKILLS
FOR MANAGEMENT

A manager is a person who continually finds mechanisms for energizing every part of the institution to accomplish the broad goals of the organization. To accomplish this end, he needs to think in terms of interacting components, formulation of objectives, strategies, and control mechanisms.

The four chapters dealing with the conceptual skills of management provide the reader with broad concepts related to the management function. The application of these concepts in actual situations enables the manager to allocate scarce resources for the accomplishment of organizational goals.

THE MANAGEMENT RESPONSE

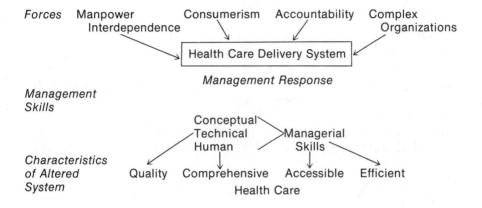

Forces   Manpower   Consumerism   Accountability   Complex
          Interdependence   Organizations

Health Care Delivery System

Management Response

*Management
Skills*

Conceptual
Technical   Managerial
Human   Skills

*Characteristics
of Altered   Quality   Comprehensive   Accessible   Efficient
System*
                            Health Care

LEARNING OBJECTIVES

After carefully reading this chapter, you will be able to:

1. State four forces in society that have an impact on health care institutions.

2. State three main types of skills needed by managers in today's health care institutions.

3. List four characteristics of the changing health delivery system.

4. Diagram the health management response model.

INTRODUCTION

The health care delivery system is in transition. Caught up by outside forces—increased government intervention; the rise of consumer demands for more accessible, comprehensive, and quality care; the need for a broader base for decision making on health care policy; the movement of health care institutions toward a more complex organizational form; and the increasing use of newly created paramedical specialties—the institutions devoted to health care are reeling from waves of change. These changes generate new organizational forms and work demands within institutions. At the very center of this rapidly evolving system, hospitals and other health agencies face new demands as they reorganize to cope with the forces impinging on them from without and the pressure for better patient care from within.

FORCES IN SOCIETY

Accountability

On every side, health institutions are faced with the notion of accountability—for patient care programs, planning, allocation of resources, and relationships with the government and other third-party payers. This accountability requires intelligent management that is responsive to the needs of the members of the institution, enlightened about the trends in the world of administration, and that responds at every level to operating problems so that situations can be altered or expanded whenever the need arises. This accountability to the people continues to grow as consumerism becomes a vital part of health care delivery.

Consumerism

More and more frequently, the consumer of health care wants a voice in the way that this service is delivered and financed. As a result, more institutions are allowing consumer groups to be represented on governing and advisory boards.

These groups are increasingly raising the need for cost containment and better insurance so that an individual's financial resources will not be completely drained by a major illness. An example of governmental response to assistance in financing health care was the passage of the Medicare and Medicaid legislation in 1965. These programs financed medical care for the elderly and the medically indigent; however, this sudden infusion of money led to a rapid inflation of health care cost. This seemingly inexhaustible source of funds brought opportunities to expand services, update old equipment and buy new equipment, increase depressed salaries, and institute a host of other developments. Unfortunately, many health care providers continued to operate in splendid isolation from one another, propagating the high cost pathway by duplicating services and failing to establish cost controls and to use the management techniques that might prevent the wastage associated with a cost reimbursed system that had a seemingly inexhaustible money supply.

Shortly after the new payment programs were implemented, Congress passed comprehensive planning legislation. Other steps to control expenditures began to be discussed. During the decade between 1965 and 1975, many attempts were made both nationally and locally to stem the tide of price inflation and system wastages caused by excess capacity (in many but not all areas), duplication, and lax cost controls.

Complex Organization

Owing to advances in medical knowledge and technology, health care institutions have developed large staffs and complicated organizations to respond to the increased demand for more comprehensive, high quality health care. The decision-making structure now encompasses the ideas of the medical staff, trustees, consumers, and employees. The role of the manager as coordinator within these health care institutions becomes more critical. No longer can major decisions be made without much study and discussion and the involvement of many groups.

Interdisciplinary Care

Concomitant with the development of complex organizations for delivery of care is the interdisciplinary approach to care of patients. The doctor can no longer be the sole provider of care; he is now dependent upon the nurse, therapist, pharmacist, dietitian, laboratory and radiologic technologist, social worker, business manager, medical record librarian, engineering and housekeeping specialists, and a host of other specialized personnel. The team approach to patient care demands highly developed conceptual and technological skills from each member of the team. This cooperative effort is further enhanced by managers, who facilitate the environment for interdisciplinary work.

The forces of accountability, consumerism, complex organizations, and interdisciplinary patient care continually affect health institutions, forcing managers to respond with more sophisticated conceptual, technical, and human skills.

POST-TEST 1–1

What are the major forces in society affecting health care institutions today? Give examples of some specific forces affecting your own organization.

MANAGEMENT RESPONSE

The workers for whom the impact of this rapid evolution in the health field is greatest are the middle-level managers—the department heads, supervisors, head nurses, and first-line managers. These people contribute to the formation of and implement policy, control costs, direct patient care, and deal with many public groups. If each individual manager gains the insights and understands the sound practices of management, the institution will be run more effectively. If supervisors do not understand the administrative process and the basic management function carried out in an interdependent system, the institution will fail to attain its goals, evidence poor cost performance, demoralize its human resources, fail to meet social responsibility and community need, and perhaps fail as an institution.

Thus, many critical decisions in the management of a health care organization are made by the department head, floor supervisor, head nurse, and administrative staff. It is this group that must respond most rapidly to the demands being placed on the health system. It is this group that must demonstrate the conceptual, human, and technical skills needed to better perform their critical role in the administration of today's hospitals and to serve as reservoirs of insight and knowledge for their assigned personnel.

Conceptual Skills

Increasingly, management people view organizations and programs within them not as isolated units but as parts of larger systems and often containing subsystems that interact with the main institution. This line of thinking is in large part the result of a trend in science to classify and describe reality in a way that helps to account for interrelationships. Electronic engineers use electrical currents from one part of a system to feed back information and provide controls for highly automatic processes. Likewise the prudent manager uses information feedback to control prior processes in order to insure effective functioning. The systems way of thinking, then, is one of the conceptual skills that can be used by managers to keep the total institution or department in view while solving specific problems.

Equally critical responsibilities of the manager are to decide what should be done, how and when it should be done, and who should do it. In order to perform these duties, the manager must have skills in establishing concrete objectives and in designing plans and strategies for carrying out these objectives. Finally, the manager must develop control mechanisms to monitor the accomplishment of the objectives.

Technical Skills

Managers are characterized by their ability to solve problems, make decisions, insure employee productivity, and analyze and understand management-labor negotiations.

Problem solving involves a step-by-step process that insures an orderly assimilation of facts so that alternative ways of reaching a decision are available. This skill demands an understanding of the entire process and continual practice in decision making.

The manager spends considerable time training his employees and upgrading their skills so that they can function effectively in the work situation. Thus the manager must have a working knowledge of the development and implementation of educational programs for employee groups.

Finally, every manager must understand employee-management bargaining dynamics in order to cope effectively with union activities while maintaining and safeguarding the rights of the worker and management.

Human Skills

The human resources necessary for the delivery of health services are innumerable. Given the manpower intensity of the industry, much management time is spent in communicating with, motivating, and relating with health personnel. These activities require expertise and sensitivity to the needs of each employee within the organization. The human skills of management are essential if the goals of the organization are to be realized. How can patients receive care unless the employees are motivated to serve others? How can plans be implemented without communication networks? Finally, how can institutions maintain their vitality without employees who feel respected and who experience a sense of satisfaction in their work?

POST-TEST 1–2

1. Give an example of a conceptual skill used by a manager.
2. Give an example of a technical skill used by a manager.
3. Give an example of a human skill used by a manager.

ALTERED DELIVERY SYSTEM

The environmental forces of accountability, consumerism, complex organization, and interdisciplinary care are affecting the health care delivery system and forcing managers of health institutions to upgrade their conceptual, technical, and human skills. This new management expertise is brought to bear in shaping a more responsive health system that can deliver high quality, comprehensive, accessible, and efficient health care.

Quality health care refers to the level of adequacy with which health needs of a particular group of people are managed according to available service guidelines or standards. These standards refer to the organizational characteristics of the health care institution, the skill level of the people providing the services, and the quality criteria developed by accrediting and professional organizations.

Comprehensive health care refers to the provision of health maintenance, primary care, restorative care, and custodial care. This concept implies that a person has a right to a full range of services to prevent disease, to detect disease and disability in its earliest stages, and to be diagnosed and treated as well as to be rehabilitated to his fullest capacities.

Accessible health care implies that services should be available to the individual at the time and place that he needs it. The individual and institutional provider must have the necessary range of services and resources to provide comprehensive services to its clients.

Efficient health care refers to the level at which health problems are met with a minimum amount of direct and indirect costs such as lost wages or nonproductive behavior.

This type of altered delivery system should be the goal of each health worker. Effecting this change in the health care delivery system will demand more sophisticated skills of the health manager.

POST-TEST 1–3

List the four characteristics of the altered health care delivery system.

SUMMARY

Rapid change is a reality for society. Nowhere is this more evident than in the health care field. Forces such as accountability, consumerism, manpower interdependence, and complex organizations are forcing managers of health care institutions to develop highly sophisticated conceptual, technical, and human skills to cope with the new environment. If managers consistently manifest quality management practice, the health care institutions will be able to deliver health care that is of high quality, comprehensive, accessible, and cost-effective.

RECAP EXERCISE 1

Draw the management response model and discuss each component of the model:

environmental forces

management skills

characteristics of altered system

REFERENCES

American Hospital Association: *Report of the Special Committee on the Provision of Health Services.* Chicago, Ameriplan Perloff Committee, 1970.

Garfield, S. R.: The delivery of medical care. *Sci. Am. 22*:15–23, April, 1970.

Haimann, T.: *Supervisory Management for Health Care Institutions.* St. Louis, The Catholic Hospital Association, 1973.

Katz, Robert L.: Skills of an effective administrator. *Harvard Business Review.* January–February, 1975.

Myers, B. A.: *A Guide to Medical Care Administration,* vol. 1. Washington, D.C., American Public Health Association, Inc., 1965.

Learning Module 2

SYSTEMS

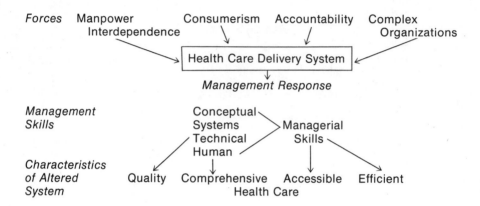

LEARNING OBJECTIVES

After carefully reading this chapter, you will be able to:
1. List the five components of a system.
2. List the four main activities of a system.
3. Identify three central problems of a system.
4. Use a system framework for defining and solving problems.

INTRODUCTION

All managers (supervisors, head nurses, department heads) need to develop and utilize concepts that will assist them in their efforts to cope with the multitude of problems which bombard them each day. A systems model that views organizations, parts of organizations, programs, and other social units as sets of interrelated and interacting parts can be used effectively by managers. This conceptual framework provides the necessary focus of attention upon the essential elements and characteristics of systems and shows how these concepts can be used to analyze problems in health care delivery.

COMPONENTS OF A SYSTEM

A system is a series of interrelated parts that function together to attain a desired goal. Health care institutions have certain *inputs* (people, money, material) that are *processed* (pulled together, rearranged, served) by people (organization, machinery) to achieve some kind of *output* (product, satisfied customer, reduction in disability). The conduct of the institution is influenced and regulated by *feedback* (information about the output) and the *environment* (forces pushing the systems in various directions). The system components are shown in Figure 1.

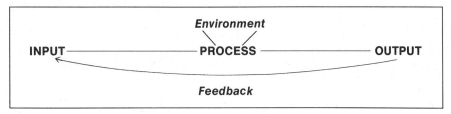

Figure 1 Systems model.

In this book, environmental forces such as consumerism, pressures for public accountability, federal legislation (e.g, national health insurance), and labor legislation influence the *inputs* that managers need to take into account as they consider how to best assemble resources to *process* them and in order to produce *outputs* — products responsive to these new and evolving demands.

✗ The manager must also be alert to the values and beliefs of those who own or control the system. For instance, the manager of a work unit in a Catholic-owned hospital would need to be sensitive to the teaching of the church, especially as it relates to such controversial issues as the right to life. Similarly, a manager of a publicly owned hospital, where there are laws and policies requiring open meetings for all decision making, would need to be sensitive about trying to establish policy or make major decisions in private meetings outside the open meetings.

Department heads and supervisors operate within the framework of organization-wide policies. Just as the overall institution manager must take account of public policies and pressures, the department head and supervisor must be sure that his or her actions are in accordance with overall organizational policy and budgets. Labor laws affect the way in which the institution operates, and union contracts and personnel policies more specifically serve as guides and rules for work-force managers.

One can benefit from viewing an organization or social unit through a systems model, since abstractions from the detail of one's own perceived reality assist one in gaining insight into the operation of a phenomenon.

All objective realities are so complex that any major attempt at detail overwhelms even the most effective managers. In almost every instance, one must use some form of abstract or conceptual model to isolate the essential elements of any problem. The systems model allows us to abstract and clearly focus upon the management function as well as its relationship to other functions (patient care, support systems, training, etc.) of a system. Furthermore, a systems model allows the manager to separate out the process of work from the materials processed and outputs achieved.

The systems model facilitates the separation of the act of production or processing from the act of controlling and coordinating all of the elements. This distinction is of great value when the people who perform the management function also perform some of the production functions. For example, nurses and physicians who provide patient care also act as supervisors and department chairmen.

The basic systems model serves to describe and analyze all types, sizes, and levels of systems. For example, the output of the health system produces certain *outcomes* in society. This can be portrayed as follows:

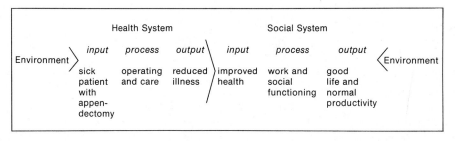

At the operating level, housekeeping provides the following example:

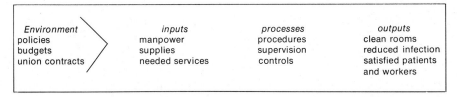

While these distinctions may seem trivial, they represent a major opportunity for managers to examine and potentially improve the functioning of their system. A contemporary example will help to illustrate this point. Medical technology now makes it possible to prolong life. This output could be characterized as a reduction of mortality. However, if the individual can never function in any normal human capacity, or perhaps never even regain consciousness or perform any productive role in society and never enjoy any discernible benefit from having been "saved," the *outcome* for society and for the individual and his family may in fact be negative.

The health care system may in this instance be criticized for producing negative benefits for the society it serves. A related question for the manager is whether devoting money and personnel to such heroic lifesaving efforts constitutes the best use of resources. Normally, first priority goes to the most critical life-saving function; however, if in having saved the life, both the individual and the larger society derive negative benefits, one must question the system.

In this example, the output of the process clearly fits within the established values and beliefs of health care systems. When the *outcome* in the larger social system comes into focus, serious questions arise as to whether the health care system should continue its usual practice without modification.

At the operating level, a problem of turnover might be initially considered as resulting from low morale. Morale is often seen as a primary function of factors associated with the work process. However, it could easily be traced to other policies outside the work process itself. For example, a hospital maintained a policy of hiring the best qualified personnel for unit management positions. Best quality was defined in part by looking primarily at number of years of education, and persons with college education were preferred. Located in a college town, this hospital was able to hire people with several years of college and often graduate students. However, this group frequently used these jobs as temporary measures to increase their income while going to school part-time or for intervals between school sessions, leaving when their short-term needs for income were met. By shifting to a policy of hiring qualified persons whose basic goals were to secure more long-term and stable employment, turnover was decreased. By examining input policies and thus redefining the problem from work practices to hiring policies, turnover was reduced.

In another case, clerks were seen to fail to supply all of the essential information for hospital records. By defining the problem as clerical error, much effort was spent on making the clerks more efficient and detailed in their responses. A young systems engineer suggested precoding all of the needed information into a checklist, thus making it easy for the clerks to record, and requiring a detailed examination. By redefining the problem, a solution was found.

POST-TEST 2–1

1. List the main components of a systems model.
2. Draw a systems model of a hospital or your department and list the various parts of each component.

ACTIVITIES OF SYSTEMS

The basic systems model can now be amplified to include other essential functions: 1) adaptation, 2) maintenance, 3) production, and 4) governance. These activities are shown in Figure 2.

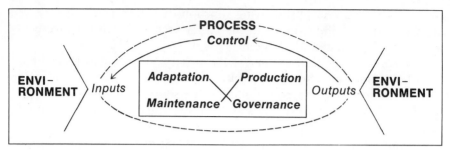

Figure 2   Activities of systems.

Adaptation

Adaptation is the system response to a change in the environment. Adaptation to change manifests itself in numerous ways in organizations. Typical organizational units concerned explicitly with change include long-range planning units and research departments. However, the need to adapt may not lead necessarily to the establishment of any specialized unit for this purpose. The nurse, the doctor, the social worker, the manager, and others in their own way keep up with changes in their fields and the changes occurring in the populations, groups, and individuals that they serve. When the environment of the organization, its clients, its ways of producing goods or services, and its products remain relatively stable, little adaptation may be required.

At the overall organizational level, long-range planning and development are two major adaptation roles. The planners seek to predict changes in client needs and technological development that might help the organization to be of better service to their clients. They study population and disease trends to keep abreast of changes in the needs of people being served. Development officers keep track of philanthropic giving and the changing patterns of financing services. Needs and interest expressed by supporters of the institution provide other guides to ways in which the organization can better serve and possible sources of funds for such services.

At the departmental and program level, managers go to institutes, attend professional meetings, keep up with professional literature and reports of new products, and exchange ideas with neighboring groups to stay abreast of trends and developments affecting their work.

Some of the changes in the health service industry that require organizational adaptation are increased governmental regulations, new therapeutic techniques, personnel licensure requirements, and increased unionization.

Maintenance/Support

Maintenance and support deal with the activities associated with providing the necessary resources for keeping the system operational.

This area involves both human and material resources. This concept also implies that an organization must maintain its basic functioning in the face of changes that are constantly occurring in the environment.

At the level of the society, health services help people to enjoy their lives and to share in the production of goods and services in exchange for income and other rewards. School systems serve to assist in socializing children for societal roles and to supply prepared persons for work roles. In the organization, personnel and training departments serve to find, train, and develop incentive systems to keep the production process supplied with qualified people. At the individual managerial level, coaching of subordinates and evaluation of performance and motivational activities help to keep production going at a satisfactory pace for both the employer and employee.

Production

The production function is concerned with the major work of the institution. In the case of the hospital, the production processes would include the diagnosis, treatment, and education of patients, the education of employees and consumers, the generation of new ideas for treating people, and the performances of appropriate community services.

For the business office, the recording of transactions, billing appropriate clients, and developing control statistics and reports constitute the production process. In the dietary department, the preparation, serving, and recycling for the next meal are basic production functions. In housekeeping, cleaning to maintain a proper environment for work and patients is the central task. For the managers of these units, keeping track of work flows, motivating people, and controlling the process are all important elements of the personal production function.

Governance

Board members in hospitals, physician-owners of group practices, stockholders and boards of business organizations, and elected officials of governments typically govern their respective areas of responsibility. Within the legal scope of their responsibilities, they establish and implement the basic purposes of the organization, set policies, and determine the overall direction of the programs. In general, this group represents the organization to others in the environment and seeks approval for its mission and for the resources needed to carry out the mission. Managers and administrators generally serve as chief executive officers to implement the policies and decisions of these governing groups.

Within such governing groups, executive committees and other groupings of board members and management work to determine in detail the directions that should be taken and when objectives and goals have been accomplished. Administrators and managers use their technical expertise to help set goals, establish and utilize control systems, monitor work performance, and manage the people by whom the goals are carried out.

At the departmental or program level, the general direction and governance of work activities are carried out by the department head, often in consultation with members of the department and in general compliance with policies and goals of the overall organization. At the unit level, supervisors also exercise governance authority but within a far more circumscribed set of rules and policies. Each level of systems, however, has some discretion or freedom of action. Lower levels of organizations typically have the least amount of authority in carrying out their mission. However, in the medical care field, unlike many others, the actual producer of care—the physician and other health professionals—have great latitude in what they may decide for their work practices and procedures.

Who decides overall policies and procedures for work? This question requires continual attention and frequently becomes the center of conflict and problems for organizations. Regulatory agencies and other governmental units set rules for organizations. Workers often organize unions to gain a stronger voice in deciding who does what work, under what conditions, how decisions about personnel will be made, and what compensation will be given. Professionals reserve the right to decide their work and procedures. When professional association pronouncements have not succeeded, some professional groups have used traditional forms of collective bargaining to further pressure organizations to recognize their right to decide certain issues.

Many of these questions and issues will be treated at greater length in later chapters. Control issues and methods, a key management task, makes up a large part of this text and is dealt with in depth in Chapter 5.

POST-TEST 2–2

1. Define the following activities of systems:
production/support
maintenance
adaptation
governance
2. Give an example of each of the above-mentioned activities within a hospital, department, nursing home, and/or health maintenance organization and for your own job work unit.

SYSTEM CONCEPTS AND PROBLEM IDENTIFICATION
Systems Problems

Goals represent a major problem for all levels of systems. At the level of society, the governing authorities must decide how to best maintain the overall social system. Resources given to health services for acute care cannot be given simultaneously to buy food, although food is a potentially greater contributor to health status. Choices must be made as to types of service systems, such as fee-for-service medicine or prepayment on a per person basis no matter how much service is used. Trade unions may prefer governmental financing for health services, whereas physicians and other providers may wish to deal directly through consumers or private agencies.

At the organizational level, some board members may prefer to support services with high prestige value (the latest technology in the field) while others may prefer economy of operation and waiting until all aspects of new technology can be proven and made available on a "pay as you go" basis. Within the professional staff, some will prefer placing emphasis on research and teaching, with less attention given to patient comfort and basic care. Others will prefer growth, placing a high priority on carving out new areas of work for the organization rather than concentrating on doing a limited number of things well and stabilizing the organization.

Decisions and choices about the basic services, who to serve, what quality of product is necessary, and how to work are but a few of the basic goal choices of organizations.

System integration and coordination represents another major problem or task for the organization. Groups and individuals must be related to one another to create a product that brings many benefits to the whole patient. The contributions of research organizations must be integrated and coordinated with basic producers of health services to insure that new knowledge is delivered to people. The work of the surgeon must be coordinated with that of the faculty practitioner and the rehabilitation worker and, as importantly, with the family and community. Within the institution, the work of dietary departments must mesh with housekeeping and with nursing. Specialists must work with administrators and supportive personnel. Admitting clerks, nursing management, and the accounting office must be closely interrelated to insure proper information flows and appropriate services and charges along with the meeting of patient care needs.

The personal needs, aspirations, and contributions must be meshed with organizational needs, demands, and reward systems. Coordination with school systems helps to insure proper preparation of workers for necessary tasks. Discharge planning, with specific needs and procedures specified, helps nursing home personnel to more appropriately receive and care for patients coming from acute care hospitals.

The world of work is filled with coordination and integration problems. Nowhere does this need seem to be a greater problem and challenge than in the health care field. While there are many specific problems in health care services, all social systems have similar problems.

Resource allocation represents a third major problem area for managers, one in which the manager claims special competence in terms of developing and applying decision rules. Given the complexity of health services, the many powerful professionals, and the size of the industry, resource allocation takes on special importance. Rarely do we have sufficient resources to do everything everyone wants to do, so decisions must be made as to how and where to allocate scarce resources. Goal conflicts ultimately result in struggles to gain control over resource allocation.

Managers must insure that all basic services and groups receive the resources they need to carry out their work and to keep the quality of group and individual contributions at a high level. In many respects, the responsibility for balancing the resource allocation of the organization among competing interest groups and needs is uniquely a manager's role. Switchboard operators may not be as powerful a group as are surgeons, but their requirements must be met or the organization faces breakdowns in vital communications. Well-established and entrenched interest may be more powerful, but new services and fledgling specialties must also be supported in order to keep up with technological advances and to maintain quality services. Managers must continually balance the interests of the new and unpowerful against those of the strong and established if the organization or department is to thrive and adapt to changing needs.

Cost increases constitute one of the most persistent problems facing the health care professional. Hospital administrators and other health care managers continue to seek improved work methods, more efficient machinery, faster and more economical processing of information, and a host of other improvements to reduce the cost of providing patient care. These and other such approaches focus principally upon the internal production process of the institution.

At the individual institutional level, these approaches constitute important contributions. However, the question must be raised as to whether other subsystems of the health care system might produce similar outcomes at lower cost. Specifically, could the client or patient do something for himself to avoid entering the high-cost health facility in the first place?

Consider heart disease as an example. Treatment for the problem in a hospital generates high cost. At the extreme, transplant surgery generates both high cost and still uncertain outcomes. At the preventive side of the spectrum, the combination of a reduction in smoking, reduced intake of cholesterol, lowered blood pressure, and lowered weight can reduce the incidence of heart disease, thus avoiding the use of resources in repairing damage and rehabilitating the patient. In general, a healthier population requires fewer resources applied to curative health services. To get at this solution, it becomes necessary to look at events and processes that occur before the patient reaches the health service.

Another example at the operating level illustrates the same point. New employees often must be trained and oriented to the specific task of the individual institution. When small numbers of people pass through for training, training proves spotty and less than adequate, leaving poorly trained employees functioning at low levels of performance and burdening superiors with a difficult task of supervision. Many hospitals and other health institutions increasingly seek the aid of vocational training schools to provide basic training to candidates *before* they come to the job. A school serving a wider community would be able both to specialize in training and to have a steadier flow of students. Persons unable to perform minimally would be eliminated from job consideration before their ineptness could endanger patients.

POST-TEST 2–3

Consider your own system level and indicate some of your problems of governance, integration, coordination, and resource allocation. What are the contending interests in each of these problem areas? Could you resolve some of these issues by reformulating the problem or changing some aspect of the system such as inputs, process, or outputs?

Systems and Objectives

Use of the systems model makes it possible to focus upon objective outputs. By specifying outputs of a system, a manager may then determine whether the overall system's performance meets expectation. As the objectives gain specificity, more precise measurement of system performance becomes possible.

Many organizations have vague or nonexistent specifications as to what they desire to achieve. High-quality care at reasonable cost often constitutes the beginning and end of the stated objectives. In other organizations, objectives can be agreed upon and established for the most trivial matters only, a situation not unlikely when conflict exists about what precise objectives should be for the use of organizational resources. It becomes impossible to determine whether objectives constitute unifying themes when attempts at greater specificity fail.

Another problem comes from implementing objective-setting management techniques as a major change in the management process. While objectives can help to order, unify, and give cohesion to an otherwise drifting organization, organized chaos may be the only result in the first few *years* of application. Also, even well-articulated objectives, brilliantly planned, executed, and evaluated, will not save an organization that has elected to compete in a glutted market or provide an unnecessary service. Careful attention must be given to defining the overall nature of one's service, how it relates to the population to be served, its differentiation from other providers, and the special niche that one plans to fill. A nursing home designed to serve a young population will work only if sufficient numbers of young people need the service developed.

Another critical issue concerns the difficulty of installing an objective-setting, implementation, and evaluating system within an ongoing operation. Like any other change, this method of managing must be carefully thought out, tested in the highest levels of the organization, and evaluated. Quick results seem unlikely when one considers the fact that the structure of the organization—its decisional processes, its human resources, and its general way of carrying out work—were designed for other modes of management. Education, trial runs, tryouts from top to bottom in the organization, and much selling, exhorting, communicating, and just plain hard work must go into a successful implementation in any setting. On the positive side, one should remember that most criticism of the health care system asserts that new breakthroughs in the delivery of health services seem likely to come from improved management of resources and not from new medical technologies.

SUMMARY

Systems concepts can be used to more effectively analyze and organize one's orientation to work and the problems encountered in improving performance. Reflection upon the changes and demands in the environment of one's immediate system and the outcomes or inputs from your system into another frequently suggests improvements and ways to solve problems not otherwise manageable or even recognized. By establishing explicit objectives, plans for their implementation, and performance standards for evaluation, one can develop a focus for attention superior to the drift frequently associated with less organized ways of managing. Significant though not insurmountable problems exist in implementing the system from the top down to the lowest system level. However, one can produce long-term results if top management personnel take and maintain prime responsibility for results.

RECAP EXERCISE 2

George Johnson has just been hired as director of housekeeping (or substitute a program or department with which you are more familiar for a department comprising 60 per cent females and 40 per cent males, the majority of whom are black. Productivity has been low and absenteeism high for some time. Area supervisors are predominantly white males. Before jumping in with any specific programs to improve work performance and morale, George is asked to do a complete assessment of the situation.

1. Sketch out some of the major system components and other aspects that George should consider in his assessment.
   a. Environmental inputs to institution
      examples: women's liberation, race relations, labor market conditions
   b. Process
      examples: personnel policies, pay practices, purchasing policies
   c. Outputs
      examples: clean rooms, safe walking surfaces
2. Consider also some of the functional characteristics of this departmental system and list some of the possible problem or opportunity areas for improvement.
   For example:
   a. Production processes
      cleaning supplies, organization of teams
   b. Supportive services
      maintenance, climate promoting people's growth and development, civil rights
   c. Maintenance
      training of people, locker facilities, dining
   d. Adaptive function
      work improvement methods, evaluation of new products, contract housekeeping
   e. Managerial
      evaluation of personnel, feedback systems for work improvement and quality control
3. Select two of the areas listed in question 2 for improvement and prepare written objectives, including:
   a. Condition requiring objective to remedy or improve.
   b. Objective — what to accomplish, how much, when, who.
   c. Critical steps necessary for change to occur.
   d. Major reasons for others to support and accept.
   e. Indicators of success.

REFERENCES

1. Ackoff, R. A.: Towards a system of systems concept. *Management Science 71*:661–671, July, 1971.
2. Carzo, Rocco, and Yanouzas, John N.: *Formal Organizations: A Systems Approach.* Homewood, Ill., Richard D. Irwin, Inc., 1967.
3. Churchman, C. West.: *The Systems Approach.* New York, Dell Publishing Co., 1968.
4. Exton, William, Jr.: *The Age of Systems.* New York, The American Management Association, 1972.
5. French, Wendell: *The Personnel Management Process,* 2nd ed. Boston, Houghton Mifflin Co., 1970.
6. Johnson, R. A., Kast, F. E., and Rosenzweig, J. E.: *The Theory and Management of Systems.* New York, McGraw-Hill Book Co., 1963.
7. Kast, Fremont E., and Rosenzweig, James E.: *Organization and Management: A Systems Approach.* New York: McGraw-Hill Book Co., 1970.
8. Katz, Daniel, and Kahn, Robert L.: *The Social Psychology of Organizations.* New York, John Wiley & Co., 1966.
9. Lawrence, Paul R., and Lorsch, Jay W.: *Organization and Environment: Managing Differentiation and Integration.* Boston, Harvard University Press, 1968.
10. United Hospital Fund of New York: *An Administrator's Survey of Systems Concept.* Englewood Cliffs, N.J., Prentice-Hall, Inc., 1971.

PLANNING AND OBJECTIVE-SETTING

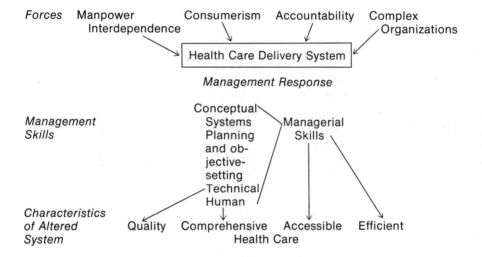

Forces Manpower   Consumerism   Accountability   Complex
      Interdependence   Organizations

Health Care Delivery System

Management Response

Management Skills   Conceptual Systems Planning and ob-jective-setting   Managerial Skills

Technical Human

Characteristics of Altered System   Quality   Comprehensive   Accessible   Efficient
                    Health Care

LEARNING OBJECTIVES

After carefully reading this chapter, you will be able to:

1. Define planning.
2. Define objective-setting.
3. Describe the manner in which planning and objective-setting interrelate.
4. Specify the levels of planning and objective setting.
5. List the five elements of the planning process.

INTRODUCTION

Managers live and work in a variety of systems. Of these multiple systems, some come under the primary jurisdiction of the manager, such as a particular department; others supply inputs or receive output for his area of responsibility, e.g., housekeeping services; and the third type represents the overall organization to which he reports. Each of these systems has objectives that it must accomplish in order to satisfy economic and human needs. Objectives for systems represent end points for achievement as well as statements of priority and interest.

Objectives also represent future states of being, activity, and accomplishment. As such, they provide useful guides for thinking about the future. However difficult it is to arrive at this statement of desired affairs, much thinking through or planning must precede action. Planning helps to progressively anticipate events necessary for achievement of objectives. It also provides the vehicle for gaining the necessary knowledge and support for achieving objectives. Not infrequently, it supplies the necessary understanding for modifying and changing objectives. Planning and objective-setting go hand in hand, since objectives provide a target for accomplishment while planning builds the necessary superstructure for accomplishment.

Planning's orientation toward the future also helps to anticipate trouble areas. How serious a barrier would one of the unwanted but possible deviations become to the accomplishment of the objective anticipated by the plan? How can the cost of such a deviation be decreased? Should some backup plan be developed to account for contingencies? Would the cost of such a backup plan outweigh the benefits to be derived from it? Thus planning and objective-setting continually interact to provide a forward movement of the organization toward desired goals.

PLANNING AND OBJECTIVE-SETTING DEFINED

Planning

A plan is a predetermined course of action that an institution follows to accomplish a certain set of objectives. A plan is a road map for reaching goals.

The need for planning stems from conditions of work, changing external and internal environments, and human limitations and concerns.

When people work alone, without affecting others, their planning needs may be neglected at some cost to themselves but without directly affecting the flow of work to others. In today's health care world, interdependencies abound. Nursing plans must mesh with physician, housekeeping, dietary, ancillary service, and related agency expectations and capabilities to sustain results achieved in the health care service. In every instance, the output or product of one unit immediately produces an input into a related system. The overall transaction between systems must be carefully considered and planned in order to achieve coordination and quality results.

As size and complexity grow, dealings among units and people become less informal and direct. Written plans, procedures, and other communications become essential to more accurately identify and specify the precise expectations and timing of events. Objectives, procedures, and evaluation criteria become clearer and more acceptable to all parties in the explication process involved in planning. Plans help people to anticipate events and to avoid continual crisis intervention, since a well-thought-out course of action specifies certain events that need to occur, when, where, and how they should occur, and who should insure their occurrence.

POST-TEST 3–1

Define planning.

Objective-Setting

Objectives are the goals or end points toward which an organization or department moves. The objectives of a hospital are patient care, education, research, and community service. The resources of the institution are organized to accomplish these objectives.

The systems model lends itself to focusing upon objective outputs. By specifying outputs of a system, a manager may then determine whether the overall system's performance meets expectations. As the objectives gain specificity, more precise measurement of system performance becomes possible.

Not only can overall systems' objectives be established with their respective performance measures or criteria, but also individual subsystem objectives can be established. Ideally, the objectives of each level of a system will complement and support the achievement of objectives of other levels of the system. For example, an objective of the dietary department to produce meals at an average cost of, say 85¢, should not sacrifice a medical and nursing objective of providing appropriate nutritional balance. In establishing objectives at any level or part of a system, due care needs to be taken to insure against a negative impact on the other systems being served.

Objectives have several major characteristics. Basically, they specify a particular state of affairs that one intends to affect or change. The plan or the desired course of events necessary to achieve the particular state of affairs also has to be specified. An objective should fully declare the outcome of the effort in terms of what one will do and how and why it will be done. An objective should result in action in pursuit of the declared intention. For example, physicians, nurses, and social service workers at an acute-care general hospital might be concerned about readmission of persons transferred to nursing homes. The basic objective might be to reduce readmissions from 15 per cent of those transferred to 5 per cent over a one-year period. The course of events to achieve this might be to perform a social, medical, and nursing workup on each patient just prior to transfer. It might also include inviting a nursing home representative to the hospital to review the case prior to moving and the development of a complete transfer record for use by the nursing home personnel in preparing and carrying out their plans. A procedure for implementing the objective, announcing its implementation, and inviting others not on the hospital staff to participate also needs to be included.

A plan, then, is a predetermined course of action that an institution follows in order to accomplish a certain set of objectives. The objectives specify a state that the institution hopes to attain.

POST-TEST 3–2

1. Define objective-setting.
2. Describe the interrelationship of planning and objective-setting.

LEVELS OF PLANNING AND OBJECTIVE-SETTING

The manager cannot set objectives and plan in a vacuum. He must be aware not only of the major goals of his own organization but also of the objectives of the national, state, and local environment in which his institution is situated. This is also true within an organization, since the manager of the x-ray department cannot set objectives and plan for events that are dissonant with the objectives and plans of the total institution.

Thus planning and objective-setting occur at many levels of organizations. At the larger system level, we find national planners concerned with ways to overcome major health problems of large numbers of people. In the battle against cancer, for instance, major strategic (long-range and general) plans exist to conduct basic research to understand and prevent or cure cancer. This involves the National Cancer Institute, cancer research centers, cancer centers where the latest techniques can be tested and demonstrated, grants to individual researchers, special grants to insure that all medical students get up-to-date information, and continuing education programs for practicing physicians. Public health education programs and other efforts go more directly to individuals and groups likely to be at high risk of contracting the disease. At local levels, major teaching centers plan to marshal their resources to attack the problems involved. At the unit level, one finds nursing and physician teams planning to utilize the latest therapies. Engineering must plan to maintain appropriate equipment, housekeeping to clean, and administration to finance and staff; and a host of other related efforts must be mounted to insure overall success of a new venture. All of these efforts must mesh for success.

Changing national health goals and objectives require shifts in local and state resource allocation and altered health plans for new health care processes. For example, as older people now constitute a larger part of the population, national policy shifts to a concern for their special needs. In a systems framework, this would lead to approximately the interrelated events depicted in Figure 3.

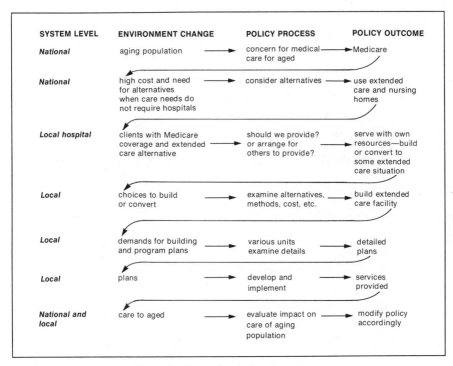

Figure 3   Interrelated planning events.

The example in Figure 3 demonstrates the fact that health systems, objectives, and plans interrelate. The way in which a specific national or state policy plan affects a given local or specific organization's operations will vary according to circumstances and choices made locally. Since national plans must cover a great variety of individual and local circumstances, they will be more general in nature with specificity increasing until at the work level, we can expect to find more definitive detail—that is, what must be done, how, when, where, and by whom. Naturally, the more definitive the objectives and plans, the more specific will be the measures you might use to evaluate the success of the plans.

POST-TEST 3–3

You are the manager of the dietary department of King's Memorial Hospital, a 300-bed facility located in an urban center. Sixty-five per cent of the people in the hospital service area are 65 or over, and many of these people do not have proper eating habits. After discussions with the people in your department, you have decided to start a "meal on wheels" program for the elderly people in the area. You think that this would meet both a patient care and community service objective for your department. Before presenting this program to the administrator for approval, how would you determine whether this program is congruent with the objectives and plans of the following groups:

1. the hospital
2. the community
3. the state
4. the nation.

ELEMENTS OF THE PLANNING PROCESS

The planning process is composed of five major elements: environmental assessment, objective formulation, program development, program implementation, and program evaluation. These activities continually interact with one another, as shown in Figure 4.

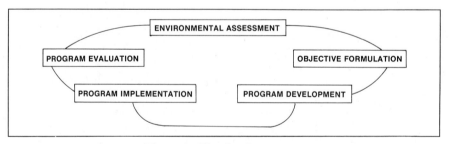

Figure 4 The planning process.

Environmental Assessment

Organizations and individuals begin to consider planning usually after some change or opportunity for change reaches a sufficiently high level of awareness. The stimulus may come from increased turnover of employees, decreased utilization of a given service, increased demand for an existing service, patient or physician dissatisfaction with results, and a host of other sources. Once aware of some need or opportunity for benefitting from planning, a purposeful assessment of environmental conditions and internal resources follows.

Such concerns apply not only to higher levels of organization but to all types of work units. Consider the problem of absenteeism in the pharmacy. When the pharmacy chief considers his organizational environment, he takes into account overall institutional policies relating to wages and fringe benefits, hiring practices, promotion policies, the climate of administration, and the interactions among his employees and other departments. An internal assessment would include studies of how work assignments, supervisory attitudes, physical conditions, and other such factors influence employee attitudes and participation. The pharmacy chief might also look at employee characteristics and how they affect absenteeism. This type of assessment contributes to a clarification of the overall goal of reducing absenteeism.

Periodic review of one's total operation provides an important opportunity both for reviewing accomplishments and for developing new objectives. In a major review, all basic functions of any system should be reviewed. Fundamental questions can be raised about the primary production process of the unit. Does every aspect of patient care, housekeeping, and radiologic services meet all of the organizationally or professionally established standards for comprehensiveness, quality, cost effectiveness, and continuity of care? Does an appropriate system exist for securing, evaluating, and utilizing the latest knowledge in the field? Are personnel well trained? Do they have up-to-date job descriptions? Is the compensation for personnel adequate in terms of internal wage structures, community wage standards, and professional standards in the field? Are there areas in which additional study might reveal new opportunities for doing your work better? Do you have established policies and internal control mechanisms which insure that you can effectively evaluate the quantity and quality of work in your area of responsibility? When more radical changes are envisioned, such as opening a new unit, all of these questions and more would need to be answered for the totally new operation. This type of analysis assists the manager in problem identification and initiation of new service programs.

Forecasting of future events from historical analysis is another dimension of environmental assessment. With forecasts in hand about the most likely future states, decisions can be made about what the organization should do to anticipate and meet these contingencies, and then objectives and programs can be developed to meet them.

Monitoring the environment provides information about the needs, problems, and opportunities of a department or an institution both at the present time and in the future. These data can then be used to develop the objectives of the plan.

Objective Formulation

The stimulus for setting objectives for improved or even radically altered performance comes from a variety of inputs to the system in which one operates. Daily concerns are a major source of objectives. Others come from radical or major changes in the overall concerns of the total system in meeting social needs.

Objectives should be specific enough to be evaluated. For example, if absenteeism is a major problem area in your department and you want to formulate an objective dealing with the reduction of absenteeism, the over-all objective statement for this area might read: "By the end of a six-month period, the absenteeism rate will be reduced by 50 per cent." This statement specifies a time frame (by the end of a six-month period) and a situation that can be measured (reduction of absenteeism rate by 50 per cent). From this main objective, sub-objectives dealing with the absenteeism rate can be formulated. They might include specific items such as instituting an orientation session with each new worker and a careful review of requirements. One objective might be to insure understanding of policy. Specific actions to accomplish this goal would include periodic follow-up sessions, written handouts on policy, occasional department-wide sessions to review policy, immediate follow-up on policy infractions to determine cause and correct problems, and other such specific actions to be planned and implemented throughout the immediate and long-range future. The decision as to which of the possible activities will stay in the planned program will depend in part upon the assessment of all alternatives to determine which of them has the greatest likelihood of success.

Furthermore, each specific objective necessary to reduce absenteeism should be assessed in terms of its relative impact on the problem. All possible actions need not be specified, but the three to five choices that are incorporated into the plan should meet the criteria of attainability, acceptability, and clarity. The end results of each objective should be expressed in terms of amount of change expected (this could be dollars lost by overtime required to perform task not completed, money saved, percentage of reduction in absenteeism, and the time frame for accomplishment). If the overall objective is to reduce absenteeism by 50 per cent, it might be achieved in part by orientation and counseling sessions to reduce 25 per cent the absenteeism that is due to lack of understanding of rules and/or supervisory attitudes and expectations of workers. The development of specificity contributes to the exactness of programs as they relate to the precise problems that must be overcome. All of these procedures contribute to the development of a complete plan, which integrates various objectives and programs and further insures an accurate evaluation of the entire program.

Program Development

After the objectives have been clearly defined, the programs will translate the objectives into action.

Decision making involves the allocation of resources among alternative solutions. For example, if a head nurse wants to improve the productivity of the nurse aides on her floor with a training program, she has many factors to consider. How will the program be staffed and organized? Should it be done in conjunction with a total program for the nursing department? Could the local vocational school do the training? Each approach has a different cost, a different set of organizational arrangements, different benefits, and different drawbacks. The optimal solution needs to be selected.

Gaining approval for the program requires a further analysis of its organization. Is it consistent with organizational policy? Were adequate data used in identifying the problem and the cost for implementing the plan? Is it understood by those involved and those whose cooperation must be secured? Does the plan fit the situation? In the development of the plan, these questions should be asked continually.

The examples used here relate to specific units, but the overall process can be and is used in the development of multiple programs. In the process of planning for one department, issues and programs that relate to other departments may arise, leading to the involvement of higher levels of the organization. Although the impetus to plan often comes from higher level expectations of departments, the flow of initiative can come from lower levels in the organization as well. This statement also holds true for single health care organizations. One institution's need for training may be shared by others, leading to a group effort to share training services or even to arrange for local school systems to conduct the necessary training for all concerned. Again, it must be emphasized that the explication process involved in planning inevitably relates to other systems, and in the process of planning for the future, one often finds solutions and problems both broadened and simplified by trying to relate the experience of one unit with those of other units in the system.

Program Implementation

Adoption of the program will require concurrence by others, often including many of those consulted in the process of developing objectives and investigating environmental problems and constraints. Before approval and acceptance are obtained, the resource requirements—personnel, money, materials, and related services and supplies—must be worked out carefully. In addition, the working relationships with others necessary for the plan's success should be specified in terms of who will be involved, what must be done and when and how to do. A training or orientation objective should be carefully discussed with the institution's director of education and director of personnel. They might be able to handle part of the work required before employees reach the work assignment as well as offer helpful suggestions and assistance in carrying out the necessary activities in the unit concerned.

Coordination and discussion among work groups, professionals, managers, consumers, and many others likely to be affected by the plans may pave the way for later acceptance and sharpen the thrust of the plan. In considering who might logically contribute to the success of your plan, it helps to refer to the systems model presented earlier. Who will supply the inputs necessary for the plan's success? What kinds of altered outcomes can be anticipated? What subsystems and adjoining systems processes will be affected by contemplated changes? If you manage a clinic and wish to rearrange the procedures for laboratory tests performed by an outside laboratory or even an "inside" laboratory under someone else's control, laboratory personnel's knowledge of the way that the plan will affect their own operation may make the difference between success and failure. Housekeepers' schedules depend upon admissions and discharge times; dietary schedules depend upon both incoming supplies and the flow of work and therapy in patient units. Coordination needs seem to increase as the number and variety of professionals affected increases in the health care world. An almost continuous effort must be made to coordinate activities, especially long-range plans for changes.

Committees also serve control purposes. Planners (and managers are planners) need to take actions to obtain feedback on how well their directives and programs serve intended needs; likewise the planner needs to ascertain how well the plan can be expected to meet the diverse needs represented in work units and related units. Discussion, questioning about consequences, and general probing provide information necessary for the management control function. Plans also require investigation, research and advice on facts, and assumptions and implications of planned action — especially in situations in which persons other than the planner have relevant skills and information. In health care organizations, the manager/planner often must rely primarily upon other health care professionals for important information and problem solutions that can be translated into organizational plans. This holds true for professionals and other workers as well as the consumers of the product or service. Data gathered from other sources should at a minimum be tested against the ideas and sources of the group likely to be affected to ascertain its fit with the local situation. This can be done by individual consultation and committee or group discussion.

Committees also serve as major communications networks to disseminate information, persuade members of the relevance of plans, and educate about changes and their implications. Since planning deals in concepts and abstractions as the primary product of the intellectual process, the normal communications channels and types of messages must be augmented to insure that everyone understands the plan. Concepts and abstractions associated with planning pose major challenges to the communications skills of the planner. The group discussion of plans not only informs the group of the concept but also helps the planner to further specify the meaning and implication of his plans. In the early stages of planning, the planner will be the prime beneficiary of the process; later, assuming that an effective plan results from the effort, the group will gain the most information from the discussion. (See also Chapter 9 for an in-depth discussion of communication.)

Committees also serve a judicial purpose. By exposing ideas and plans early, all parties involved are given the opportunity to insure that their needs and aspirations gain (or at any rate suffer the least) from impending changes. The committee process may work best in situations in which the plans lead to the enhancement of all of the interests involved. While the industry continues in an expansion phase and each new plan brings forth new activities and resources, committees serve this function well. Less certain success from committees can be expected when the plans lead to a situation in which what one person or group gains, another clearly loses. Bargaining, mediation, and some forms of third-party assistance may be indicated when some of the interests represented in the plan clearly derive no benefit from the plan. Regional planning agencies represent this type of third force in the allocation of roles (and thus of resources) to help the institution to grow and serve the community. Internally, progressively higher level committees decide upon allocations affecting internal units.

Program Evaluation

At the end of a specified program, an assessment should be made to determine how fully the objectives were realized. The results of the evaluation of specific programs then determine to what extent the overall plan has been effective.

This information is fed back into the environmental assessment and the planning and objective-setting cycle begins again.

In general, the environmental assessment, objective-setting, implementing, and evaluation process can be viewed as a series of interacting systems as depicted in Figure 5.

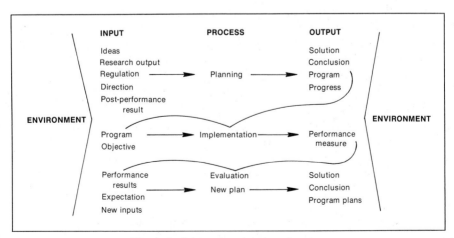

Figure 5 Interactive planning elements.

POST-TEST 3–4

Define the five elements of the planning process.

SUMMARY

Managers seek direction from their assessment of organizational policy and community need and also contribute to both by targeting future states for the organization to achieve. Plans should clarify the objectives of the group and the means for their achievement. This clarification process creates new directions for the organization to pursue and highlights opportunities to further improve performance and the overall satisfaction of the organization's members and clients.

Planning is not done in a vacuum but occurs at different levels of an institution, in the local region, the state, and the nation. In order for objectives of a hospital department to be realized, they must be congruent with those of the institution and the surrounding environment.

The planning process is continuous and includes five main elements: environmental assessment, objective formulation, program development, program implementation, and program evaluation.

RECAP EXERCISE 3

You are the director of nursing service of a 300-bed hospital. Recently you and your nursing administrative staff have decided to initiate a nursing audit. The medical staff of the hospital has developed a sophisticated medical audit program. The director of medical records has already volunteered to assist the department of nursing with this program. The administrator of the hospital has approved budgetary appropriations for a training program to introduce the nursing audit. There is a university in the area with a department of nursing. The hospital has a sophisticated computer system that has already incorporated the data-processing requirements of the medical record department.

1. Define the factors in the national, state, and local environment that affect this situation.

2. Define the objectives of the nursing audit program.

3. Develop a nursing audit program.

4. Develop an organizational plan for implementing the nursing audit program.

5. Develop an evaluation plan for the nursing audit program.

REFERENCES

1. Donnelly, Paul R.: *Guide for Developing a Hospital Administration Policy Manual.* St. Louis, Catholic Hospital Association, 1974.
2. Drucker, Peter T.: *Managing for Results.* New York, Harper & Row, 1964.
3. Drucker, Peter T.: *The Age of Discontinuity: Guidelines to Our Changing Society.* New York, Harper & Row, 1969.
4. Ewing, D. W. (ed.): *Long Range Planning for Management.* New York, Harper & Row, 1972.
5. Granger, C.: The hierarchy of objectives. *Harvard Business Review 42*:63, 1964.
6. Koontz, Harold, and O'Donnell, Cyril: *Principles of Management.* New York, McGraw-Hill Book Co., 1972.
7. LeBreton, P. P., and Henning, D. A.: *Planning Theory.* Englewood Cliffs, N. J., Prentice-Hall, 1961.
8. McConkey, D. D.: *How to Manage by Results.* New York, American Management Association, 1967.
9. Odiorne, G. S.: *Management by Objectives.* New York, Pitman, 1965.
10. Perrow, Charles: The analysis of goals in complex organizations. *American Sociological Review 26*:854–866, December, 1961.
11. Reddin, W. J.: *Effective Management by Objectives: The 3-D Method of MBO.* New York, McGraw-Hill Co., 1971.
12. Reinke, William A. (ed.): *Health Planning: Qualitative Aspects and Quantitative Techniques.* Baltimore, Johns Hopkins University Press, 1972.

STRATEGY

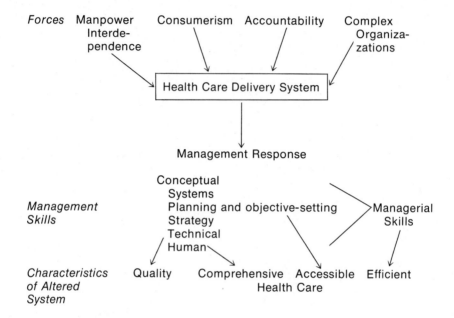

LEARNING OBJECTIVES

After carefully reading this chapter, you will be able to:
1. Define strategy.
2. Define the four elements involved in strategy formation.
3. List the five characteristics of effective strategies.
4. Discuss the role of power and influence in strategy development.

INTRODUCTION

In order for health care organizations to best serve the patients, the employees, the physicians, and the community, the organization and each hospital department must find a balance between individual resources and interest and the demands and resources of the environment. For the hospital, this means assessing the resources of the community, the medical practitioners, and the governmental and private agencies that purchase hospital services. For a department it means finding out exactly what can be accomplished using internal resources of the institution. Based on an assessment of what can be accomplished in the community to improve health and of the resources available to do the job, an organization can shape long-range goals to serve as a focal point for directing effort. After the goals have been developed, a strategy or way of proceeding can be formulated to carry out the goals.

As the organizational character emerges, its special or potentially favorable position in the environment becomes clear. For example, it does not seem far-fetched to imagine that a medical group would possess more expertise than a non-health agency in dealing with and gaining influence in the more complex bureaucratic organizations such as Professional Service Review Organizations. The medical group and its management will be familiar with medical and other quality considerations that are frequently at the center of such regional decision-making organizations. The more comprehensive the character of the organization's membership, the greater will be the likelihood that the group will be considered the logical leader in defining the needs for health services in the area.

DEFINITION OF STRATEGY

Strategy is the mechanism that the manager chooses to translate objectives and plans into reality. It is the underlying rationale for the accomplishment of goals. Gaining a well-articulated position that serves to direct the overall conduct of the institution constitutes a strategy. Strategies serve to relate goals to specific policies and programs in order to achieve a strong control thrust for the organization.

For the community hospital, the general goals of patient care, research, and education often serve as a general starting point for role definition. In a community of older persons, patient care might further be focused on problems of aging, with research in geriatrics and/or rehabilitation. Educational programs might be concentrated around the special concerns of older people and include rehabilitation, home care, and ambulatory care aids. In this case, the institution selects its most natural environmental opportunity for service. It would select and attract professionals with special concerns in this area. By concentrating its resources upon the concerns of older people, its energies and special opportunities could be used to the greatest advantage. Such a move would constitute a cohesive strategy for giving direction to the overall goals of the organization and would contribute to the development of policies and plans for its implementation.

Such a strategy represents a deliberate effort to concentrate on the problems of the major population being served. Although obstetric and pediatric services might also be offered, little opportunity would be provided to develop research and education in these areas. In other words, the strategy to concentrate on a specialized area—and a most appropriate one in view of its natural market—would serve as a guide to the allocation of resources and energy of management.

A hospital located in an area where the population composition has shifted from a wide age spectrum to a narrow (in this case, older) age range, might, as some hospitals have done, choose to move to an area where it could continue to offer a wide range of service or even to develop a new operation in another area while making the original operation more specialized to meet local needs.

Every manager in some way operates within the constraints and opportunities of his environment. In the situation cited above, the manager of obstetrics and pediatrics would probably focus attention on low cost and efficient and flexible service. Opportunities for innovation would probably revolve around flexible staffing and facility utilization. In the rehabilitation unit, however, the manager would have opportunities to develop innovative educational programs and to work out new ways of providing continuous service between units within the hospital and between the doctor's office and the home. The department manager's strategy would in essence be influenced by and fit within the overall strategy of the institution. To a large extent, however, opportunities exist for each department to develop components of strategy that also reflect the resources and interest of the unit that may not clearly fit within the overall picture. In general, the strategy of departments can be expected to reflect the overall strategy of the institution over time. One must consider, however, that the transition to a population of primarily older people does not occur overnight and that the rehabilitation department was probably at some point as constrained as the obstetrics department.

Managers at all levels of organization need to concern themselves with long-term goals and objectives that can be related to one another to provide a cohesive picture of the central thrust of the institution or department in order to guide policy and day-to-day operations. This central objective should take into account environmental and internal resources, both present and attainable. Organizations may function without an operating strategy, but they are not likely to achieve excellence in using opportunities and resources to the greatest advantage.

In planning strategy, the manager also has to keep in mind the network of interrelationships that characterize organizations and that need to be considered as strategic objectives change. These networks are visualized in Figure 6.

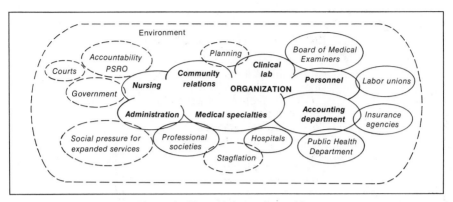

Figure 6 Network interrelationships.

The key tasks for the manager of a system are to find the combination of opportunities that should be pursued in order to gain acceptance by and utilization of resources from the systems served by his unit and to motivate system participants to perform at an optimum level. The linking together of priority goals and objectives to policies that guide actions necessary to achieve the unit's long-term goals constitutes a strategy.

POST-TEST 4–1

1. Define a strategy.
2. What is the relationship of strategy to planning and objective-setting?

ELEMENTS OF A STRATEGY FORMATION

Strategy formation is built upon several key elements. These are environmental constraints, input, process, and output factors. How these factors interact is also contingent upon power relationships among affected individuals and groups. The interaction of these elements is shown in Figure 7.

Environmental Constraints

In order to develop an effective strategy for implementing objectives and plans, the forces in the environment that hamper this process have to be known. Constraints deal with the resources, regulations, attitudes of people, technology, and cultural trends in the environment.

What kind of financial, credit, or investment policy will the organization decide is necessary? Neither the policy nor the strategic thrust can be evaluated unless the community, state, and national environment oppor-

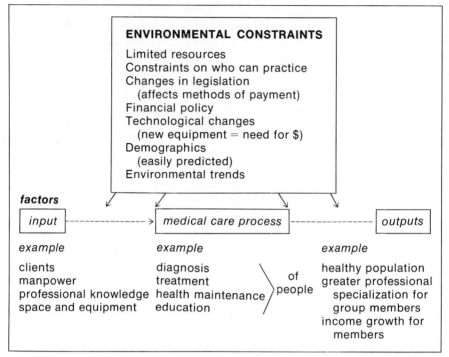

Figure 7   Elements of strategy formation.

tunities and constraints are analyzed. There are various ways in which the internal resources and environmental factors can be matched, but the organization must demand the commitment of organizational members to the specific choice. The professional is already committed to the concept of his profession. He must also be committed to business and management goals and policies to give better financial viability to his work.

Input Factors

The input elements refer to the clients' knowledge of human and capital resources that are necessary to carry out the mission of the institution. If the manager is not aware of the raw materials available, he cannot accomplish specific objectives. In order to determine the input factors that should be considered in strategy formation, the following questions should be asked:

1. *Who are the clients?* For a hospital, this would be the population in the service area, classified by age, socioeconomic status, and health profile. For a department manager, the client group could be the employees of the hospital (i.e., the personnel department), or the patients who are admitted to the hospital or nursing home (i.e., a nursing station). Sensitivity to the client group is important because different clients are approached in different ways. For example, if the organization agrees to

serve only an aged population, it may be necessary to recruit geriatric specialists and to own nursing homes and other long-term care facilities. Members of the institution may need to contact community agencies concerned with senior citizens to provide services and coordinate efforts.

2. *What are the characteristics of the system's manpower?* The organization's resource-base assessment for policy decisions must also include the personalities of physicians, administrators, and trustees involved. When a person is invited to join the organization, much thought must be given to his specific skill and how it will affect expansion or contraction of service. His personal habits, time off, dedication, and need within the community for his resources will ultimately influence organizational policy. If a physician's area of work requires new equipment, financial policy may change. Even changing demographics in the community may signal the need for new members with skills not at present included in the organization.

3. *What capital resources are necessary for the operation of the system?* In order to carry out the goals of an organization, assessment of specific capital resources such as space and equipment is needed. In order to perform surgical operations, specially equipped operating rooms removed from the rest of the hospital are essential. For the continual financing of the operation, various strategies have to be developed. It may be decided to rely less on government reimbursement, or the organization may enter new markets to maintain some combination of public and private financing. The financial policy of the organization may need revamping.

Process Factors

In determining strategy, a close examination of the organization's activities is in order. What does an institution or department need for production, maintenance adaptation, and support in delivering health care? Methods of accomplishing goals must take these factors into consideration.

Output Factors

A strategy does not take into consideration only a few resources and process variables; it goes a step further and specifies where the organization shall go and what it shall become. In other words, a strategy defines the central goal of the organization. It defines its output in order that it may realistically assess the past and current resources that provide the base for the desired new direction. Pursuing outputs that would be wasteful of community health resources or would merely satisfy the vanity of some individuals while lowering overall quality of care would constitute a breach of community trust, an unethical move for professionals. Professionals will continue to maintain community goodwill and support only so long as our actions keep the community welfare uppermost.

Strategic plans join the "might be" with the "can do" and "how to." Workable strategies reflect a reasoned relationship to opportunities and problems along with a close relationship to organizational resources, both extant and potential. The overall strategy will usually find acceptance from clients, organization managers, professionals, and board members. It should also provide a stimulus to action by all of these parties. Once the elements of strategy formation are understood, the manager interrelates these elements in the final definition of a strategy.

POST-TEST 4–2

Define the four elements involved in strategy formation.

CHARACTERISTICS OF EFFECTIVE STRATEGIES

Effective strategies have certain characteristics:

1. A strategy usually constitutes *long-term* as opposed to short-term or tactical directives. The time frame for a workable strategy will usually be about four to five years, with longer range aspirations expressed in more general terms. For instance, a strategy that seeks an increase in the involvement of the community in the overall policies of the institution might have as a corollary tactic the establishment of a community advisory committee to an alcoholic clinic. Such a move would develop a knowledge of how the clinic and the overall organization unit might work better with community groups and satisfy the insistent local pressures for direct involvement while retaining the option of determining precisely how the long-term organization would develop.

2. An effective strategy must be precise both in words and in works. Relationships among goals, policies, plans, and actions need to be clear if others besides the key formulator are to have the opportunity to participate fully in their accomplishment.

3. A strategy should have a definable relationship to organizational strengths, resources, and environmental constraints. This should be equally true with today's resources as with the resources and environmental opportunities projected for the future.

4. The strategy should be developed within a framework of acceptable risk for both the organization and its key leadership. A strategy that would leave the community devoid of its most basic health services could constitute an unacceptable risk. Investing in some highly specialized services while allowing resources to be drained from basic services necessary to meet minimal standards of accreditation could constitute both unacceptable risk for the community and a breach of professional responsibility to serve the community.

5. An acceptable strategy will achieve a viable balance between resources and professional and community interest. It will reflect the personal values of those most responsible for achievement, including trustees, key managers and medical and other staff members. It should also fit within the overall goals and objectives for the region in which the institution is located, with third-party payers and planning agencies concurring, if not actually directly approving. The same general precept applies to unit strategies within organizations, even though concurrence from outside agencies may not be necessary.

POST-TEST 4–3

List the five characteristics of an effective strategy.

ROLE OF POWER AND INFLUENCE IN STRATEGY DEVELOPMENT

In organizations in which multiple goals exist and the knowledge and skills necessary for successful functioning reside in more than a single individual, the development of consensus and agreement will be a necessary part of strategy development. Health care organizations perform many tasks that depend on the skill and knowledge of a variety of individuals. Research, education, patient care, and other goals exist side by side, with strong advocates for each pursuing the limited resources for their particular interest. Each of these goal sets represents a critical and important function of health care organizations and should be encouraged. However, the prudent manager recognizes that balance among these must be achieved and that to do so, constant attention must be directed to making sure that sufficiently strong coalitions of individuals, groups, and organizations protect and nurture each of the major goal areas.

Often organizations will pursue seemingly conflicting goals simultaneously. If sufficient resources exist, this situation can be both possible and desirable. Consider, for example, the many unknowns surrounding cancer. Should any given line of research be excluded at this time? Should health maintenance organizations be allowed to immediately displace or replace the current patient-doctor-hospital system and other provider systems of delivering care, or should we move more slowly until more can be learned of the effects of such systems compared with current practice? Some group practices currently have both prepaid clients and fee-for-service clients, thus providing experience with both forms of financing and practice.

Power and influence may be defined as the ability or potential ability to select goals and to make changes in order to attain the goals of a system. Some students examining social organizations and strategic policies see power as being possessed by a relatively small number of people and organizations. Others contend that power remains diffuse and is spread over many organizations and individuals. When an issue or policy affects the vital interests of many people and groups, attempts to influence the issue bring many more persons into the process than when the issue either has very little effect on most people or meets with general approval as being within the range of acceptable policy. Most health administrators act as if many people have power and can at least veto actions if not stop their very development.

In strategy development, the following general attributes of organizations should be considered:

1. Choices involve many interests and groups and generally represent incremental changes from the status quo.
2. Only a few of all possible policy alternatives get considered, and these represent small changes.
3. Only a few of the many possible consequences of any alternative usually receive consideration and examination.
4. Objectives are adjusted to suit the organization's usual way of accomplishing them as often as the means of carrying out objectives are modified to fit the objectives.
5. Problems and objectives get reformulated and changed as data are examined.
6. Analysis and evaluation occur sequentially, resulting in policy that evolves from a long series of amended choices.
7. Frequently, analysis and evaluation begin with a negatively perceived situation rather than an established or positively oriented goal.
8. Policy analysis and evaluation take place throughout the organization in a relatively fragmented fashion.

The improvement of strategy development, assuming that these assumptions are correct, depends heavily upon an understanding of the process that leads to strategy.

Who should be considered for involvement in strategy development? Generally speaking, those who have a major stake in the outcome and choices made *and* the opportunity and power to modify or veto the outcome should be consulted. Assuming that some interests, such as the medical staff, have major representative structures, one can look to persons in formal positions of power. Coalitions often develop around issues and programs with more informal leadership, and these should be identified and sounded out on their concerns.

Persons and groups with "power" need to be considered at some point in the strategy development process. One may view the question of power by asking who has the control or use of resources needed by others to carry out their operations. For instance, the travel budget for an organization may be controlled by an administrator to whom a department head or supervisor reports. This control over a necessary resource provides the administrator with control or power over those who wish to employ this resource to further their own objectives. Generally, one can expect that the administrator will allow the use of these funds when and if he perceives that their use contributes to goals and objectives thought by him to further the larger purposes of the organization.

Some resources can be used for more than one purpose. A travel budget provides less flexibility than a discretionary fund that can be used for any purpose deemed important by the controller of the fund. Also, one can reasonably expect that the diversity and overall level of resources available to the organization will contribute to the complexity and extensiveness of the exchanges that might occur within the system. A department head with a large staff can deploy his resources to achieve many purposes; one who functions alone has only his own time to allocate. In situations where most members of the overall system share similar values and expectations about goals, a wide diversity of resources can be brought to bear on any given problem or opportunity; where distrust or conflict of goals exists, exchanges and cooperation will be fewer. In determining who needs to be included in the strategy development, one must continually ask how many and what specific groups of persons have the resources that must be harnessed to make the strategy effective.

More than just money may become a valuable resource in strategy development and implementation. The following list suggests the types of resources that one might consider.

1. Money constitutes one of the resources that can be used in a variety of ways.
2. Control over jobs and assignments provides the power to determine what work and planning shall be done.
3. Control over communications channels and media provides opportunities to give visibility to ideas and shape opinion and choice.
4. Social status can affect the way that other people view and accept ideas and plans.
5. Professional knowledge and technical skills provide the necessary sources to perform many types of work, and licensing laws and institutional norms reserve many areas of choice to a few professions or specialists within them.
6. Personal popularity and admiration by others often provide the necessary extra ingredient in finding the person who will be most likely to influence others within a particular group.
7. Law and regulation limit decisions to certain professions and planning agencies, making it necessary to have their support.
8. Solidarity and cohesiveness within a group are important factors.
9. Social access to community, professional, and political groups may exist because of marriage, family, or other relationships not related to work.

10. Commitment of followers and control of organizations may go well beyond the normal allegiance associated with a work contract or understanding.

These resources will be of varying value, depending on the individual circumstances. At the outset, someone must get an issue or idea identified and accepted as meaningful to the organization. Often a critic or planner will identify and propose an area of opportunity or problem that has great consequences for the organization. An organization that wishes to have its clients value the highly personalized care will be motivated to reconsider its overall strategy and position if strong criticism about impersonality comes from persons whose opinions are highly valued.

An admissions officer may recognize problems occurring in patient care but will need to get information and feedback of his perceptions from a variety of sources to "document" his case. If agreement can be obtained that this is an important issue, more resources can be gained to study the problem fully and develop potential lines of action. In this instance, the relevance of the issue would vary among different department heads, professionals, and administrators. The medical staff would become interested if complaints came back to them from patients; similarly, nursing would be concerned, along with the x-ray and laboratory departments, with less interest coming from the housekeeping, engineering, and dietary staffs. Those who perceive their interest to be affected will be likely to attempt to exert influence in the selection of alternatives and action programs adopted to bring the reality more in line with the institution's policy. Some will wish to retain the status quo; others may desire changes in activities other than their own and perceive themselves as part of the solution rather than the problem. A department or group that possesses power resources may be uninterested in the issue and contribute little to its resolution, or the resources may not be flexible enough to apply in the particular situation.

Strategy development involves a number of stages that affect the types of resources which might be mobilized and also the influence that any given type of resources might command. The complex process of strategy development may be broken down into the following categories: initiation of the idea, staffing and planning for its development, communication, policy or organizational choice, organization of coalitions, financing, sanction, and control. At each stage of this process one can envision the kinds of resources that could be used to gain power or control.

In the case cited previously, the admissions officer may be the individual who perceives the need to consider the institution's strategy and policies related to giving personalized care. He may not, however, be the most likely person to persuade the organizational hierarchy to consider this issue. He may choose to provide data and information to his administrator as well as to give his perceptions of the situation to some of the more influential administrators, nursing directors, or physicians who come to him with complaints or suggestions. The issue may also be presented to the in-service educators or suggested to administration for discussion at an appropriate medical staff meeting. These suggestions apply when other parts of the institution need to take action. Action within the admitting department may be contained primarily within the department, so that although the administrator needs to be informed, much of the planning and strategy can be accomplished within the unit with resources at the command of the admitting officer.

When selecting persons to work out the alternatives and action plans involved, the initiator has opportunities to choose people with the requisite knowledge, skill, and reputational resources to get a fair hearing and acceptance of the ideas presented. One would not wish to select for this task a person who had a poor relationship with those who must ultimately approve or reject the idea.

Communications and the way in which an idea can be conveyed to others offer additional opportunities for getting the desired message to the appropriate people. A public relations officer or even an administrator's secretary who keeps the agenda for meetings and assists the administrator in developing communications on developments in the institution can be an important asset in getting issues highlighted.

Once an idea is accepted by those in immediate command of the situation, its fate may still rest upon what other groups think of it. It may seem perfectly logical to ask admitting office personnel to escort patients to various services in order to maintain an ongoing relationship, but if this means transferring work formerly done by orderlies or aides from other units, the affected workers individually or their union representative may find ways to effectively block or delay implementation. Similarly, some groups of the medical staff may find reasons to object to what has been proposed. In thinking through your approach, such possible objections should be considered and dealt with appropriately.

In addition, consideration should be given early to those who might most effectively organize a coalition of power-holders who can be expected to be interested in the issue at hand. The person who interacts with influential people in the more important groups is likely to be in the most advantageous position to arrange the appropriate trade offs among varying interests and line up the coalition behind the idea. Administrators and key physicians frequently act as brokers among various powerful interest groups and know how and when they might coalesce around a program.

Those who control the resources for financing or staffing a program hold considerable power over its fate. Key health agency committees controlling the budget—both capital and operating—can be expected to have a great deal of influence over strategies requiring redirection of money flows.

One must consider whether any given program thrust will result in cooperation and participation by those who must act to carry out the program. Will the patients accept the idea? Will physicians who refer patients participate and be supportive? Will the union go along?

Finally, one's own personality and that of persons involved in the strategic formation process can be a source of influence and power. Intelligence, sociability, friendliness, and tact can all affect how others will view and accept information and guidance from an individual. Communications and bargaining skills, discussed at great length in this book, can be important personal resources in getting the job done.

POST-TEST 4–4

1. Discuss the role of power and influence in strategy development.
2. List your most important power resources.

SUMMARY

Health care organizations and units composing them operate within environmental constraints with resources that must be thoughtfully deployed to achieve the greatest benefit. Organizational goals reflect in great measure a careful assessment of environmental opportunities and internal resources and the most advantageous match between them. The strategic goal guides manpower, financial, and other resource allocation policies, which serve to further direct day-to-day decisions and program operations.

A strategy may be viewed as the central theme or personality of the organization. When clearly articulated, it serves as a beacon light to guide the energies of the many participants in the organization and their various clientele. A strategy usually reflects the balance of power and influence both within the organization and among the organizations that regulate, seek service, and finance the operation. Shifting coalitions of participants and changing external and internal factors keep strategies dynamic but continuously long-range in nature.

A strategy by nature remains somewhat general, allowing for variations at different levels of organization and especially within various functions that make up complex health care organizations. The manager who understands strategy and can both assess the overall organizational strategy and develop a complementary strategy gains a position that can greatly enhance effectiveness in gaining resources and making contributions.

RECAP EXERCISE 4

Every organization and unit within the organization has certain central characteristics, which we might call a strategic profile. From this central theme, one can discern the way that the unit will relate to others in the organization and the clients served and the quality of the service provided. This character profile may also represent an aspiration rather than reality. Try in one paragraph to describe your own central thrust. In this statement describe how you wish to serve the organization, related departments, the clients or patients, and the people who work in the department.

Try to make this a statement of aspiration and then outline the issues that must be faced in order to achieve the overall strategic position. After doing this, go through the list of resources that might be pulled together and the people who might need to be involved at some stage of your strategy development process in order to achieve the aspiration.

REFERENCES

1. Appley, Lawrence A.: *Values in Management.* New York, American Management Association, 1969.
2. Bennis, Warren G., Benne, Kenneth D., and Chin, Robert: *The Planning of Change.* New York, Holt, Rinehart and Winston, Inc., 1969.
3. Blau, Peter M., and Richard, Scott W.: *Formal Organizations.* San Francisco, Chandler Publishing Co., 1962.
4. Brown, R. E.: *Judgment in Administration.* New York, McGraw-Hill Book Co., 1966.
5. Carlisle, Howard M.: *Situational Management: A Contingency Approach to Leadership.* New York, American Management Association, 1973.
6. Chandler, A. D.: *Strategy and Structure.* Cambridge, Mass., The M.I.T. Press, 1962.
7. Hardwick, Clyde T., and Landeryt, Bernard T.: *Administrative Strategy and Decision Making.* Cincinnati, Southwestern Publishing Co., 1966.
8. Newman, William H., and Summer, Charles E., Jr.: *The Process of Management: Concepts, Behavior and Practice.* Englewood Cliffs, N. J., Prentice-Hall, Inc., 1971.
9. Simon, Herbert A.: *Administrative Behavior,* 2nd ed. New York, The Macmillan Co., 1957.
10. Zald, Mayer N. (ed.): *Power in Organizations.* Nashville, Vanderbilt University Press, 1970.

Learning Module 5

CONTROL

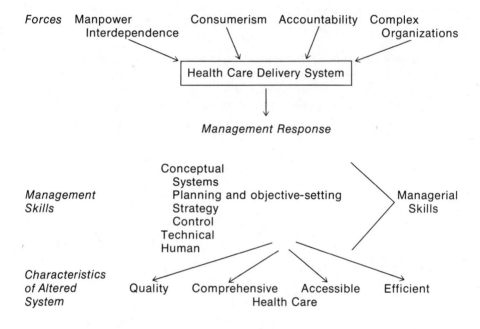

Forces Manpower   Consumerism Accountability Complex
        Interdependence   Organizations

Health Care Delivery System

Management Response

Management Skills

Conceptual
Systems
Planning and objective-setting
Strategy
Control
Technical
Human

Managerial Skills

Characteristics of Altered System

Quality   Comprehensive   Accessible   Efficient
Health Care

LEARNING OBJECTIVES

After carefully reading this chapter, you will be able to:
1. Define the control function.
2. Name the four elements of environmental assessment.
3. List the three elements of process assessment.
4. Define the three elements of product assessment.
5. Discuss the use of the budget as a monetary control mechanism.
6. Define four manpower control mechanisms.
7. Define two mechanisms for monitoring work flow.
8. Discuss the necessary factors for implementation of a control system within your area of responsibility.

INTRODUCTION

Controls are necessary for monitoring the internal and external environment, determining whether the work processes are congruent with the goals of the organization, and assuring that the final product of the organization is of high quality.

Conformity to established standards and policies serves to coordinate organizational processes, correct broken communication channels, pinpoint inefficient support services, and monitor the progress of patient care programs. Adequate control, then, depends upon a flow of significant, accurate, and timely information that monitors discrepancies between actual performance and established standards.

Today's health manager employs large numbers of personnel, coordinates the flow of patients with complicated physical and emotional conditions, and relates to a variety of professional and civic groups. Without adequate control systems, the manager is unable to monitor the allocation of resources and the accomplishment of plans and objectives.

The present era is marked by rapid changes in technology, governmental influence, and social involvement. The health manager needs monitoring mechanisms to evaluate these environmental forces and take action within the institution to adapt.

THE CONTROL FUNCTION

Definition

A management control system encompasses the policies and procedures that assist the manager in establishing goals, measuring progress, and taking corrective action. It includes the delineation and provision of environmental, process, and product assessment. An illustration of the control function is seen in Figure 8.

In order for control function to be effective, it should be forward-looking, objective, meaningful, and timely. By being forward-looking, it anticipates potential sources of deviation from standards before the deviations occur. Objectivity implies that the control system is free of the biases

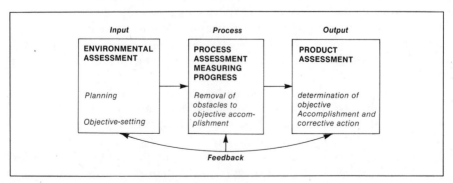

Figure 8 The control function.

of the people using it. The system also needs to be understood and accepted by those who will administer it, and finally it should be timely; that is, the reporting of deviations from standards should occur shortly after the event has happened, in terms that are understandable.

POST-TEST 5–1

1. Define the control function.
2. List the three elements of the control function.

A discussion of the elements of the control function—environmental, process, and product assessment—follows.

Environmental Assessment

The environmental assessment pinpoints the needs, problems, and opportunities surrounding the institution. The information collected then becomes the data base for the overall plan of the institution. The institutional plan, with its objectives and programs, should also specify acceptable levels of performance, which in turn become the standards for the control function.

For example, environmental assessment may clarify the need for a better system of scheduling patients in the outpatient department. Within the plan to improve patient care, an objective is formulated to insure that patients in the outpatient department will not have to wait more than 15 minutes to receive treatment. The criterion (no wait over 15 minutes) is already written into the objectives and can be used to monitor this activity.

Environmental assessment, then, encompasses the determination of needs, problems, and opportunities related to the institution and its goals and the definition of standards that show whether the objectives have been accomplished. This environmental assessment process is shown in Figure 9.

Consider the following example of environmental assessment. The personnel office has discovered an increase in the number of employee accidents in the housekeeping department (determination of a problem). To improve this condition, the personnel director and the director of housekeeping decide to develop a departmental orientation program for new housekeeping workers (strategy). The objectives for this program are

DETERMINATION OF NEEDS,
OPPORTUNITIES, PROBLEMS

DEFINITION OF GOALS
AND OBJECTIVES

STRATEGY FORMULATION

DEFINITION OF STANDARDS

Figure 9   Environmental assessment.

written in such a way that the standards of performance are included in the statement:

At the end of a six-month period and after completion of the House-keeping Job Orientation program, the employee accident rate for the Housekeeping Department will be below 10/1000 man-days of work.

Thus the control process begins with the formulation of objectives and well-defined standards (at the end of a six-month period . . . accident rate will be below 10/1000 man-days of work).

Successful environmental assessment is dependent upon relative information about the needs and problems of the institution and specific objectives and performance standards.

POST-TEST 5–2

1. Define the four elements of environmental assessment.
2. Write an objective that contains a performance standard.

Process Assessment

Process assessment insures that the objectives that have been defined are translated into workable programs with specified progress control

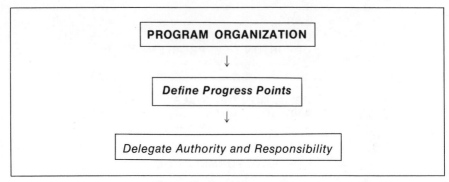

Figure 10   Process assessment.

points. Control can then be exercised during the implementation of programs, so that corrections are made immediately in programs that are not meeting objectives.

The activities of process assessment include translating objectives into programs, defining progress points for monitoring the programs, and delegating authority and responsibility for carrying out the program. These activities are shown in Figure 10.

To continue with the example of the housekeeping orientation program, the objectives (at the end of a six-month period and after completion of the Housekeeping Job Orientation program, the employee accident rate will be below 10/1000 man-days of work) relating to the program are translated into the organizational components of the orientation program. Such elements as the selection of the instructor, a room for the session, and the content to be covered have to be considered. Along with these factors, the housekeeping manager has to decide how the employees will know about the program. All of these points need to be considered when organizing programs that flow from objectives.

Following from this process, certain dates during the presentation of the program are then specified for checking that the program content is being covered and people are attending (define progress points). Finally, authority and responsibility are delegated to the staff development people to implement the program (delegate authority and responsibility).

Process assessment thus begins with a well-organized program for each objective and proceeds to the delineation of progress points so that the program can be monitored while it is operational and finally to delegation of authority and responsibility to others to carry out the program.

POST-TEST 5–3

Define the three elements of process assessment.

Product Assessment

The final phase of the control process involves the comparison of completed action with established standards, the decision as to whether objectives have been met, and the taking of corrective action if performance falls short of objectives. The sequence of events for product assessment is shown in Figure 11.

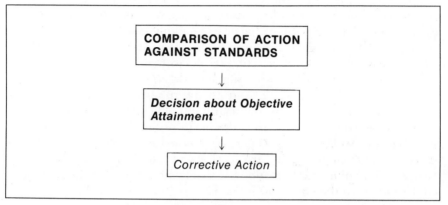

Figure 11   Product assessment.

Continuing the example of the housekeeping orientation program, the accident rate for the housekeeping employees is calculated six months after the orientation program and then compared with the standard of a 10/1000 man-days (comparison of action with standards). If the accident rate is lower, the objectives of the orientation program have been accomplished (decision about objective attainment). A decision is then made by the director of housekeeping about the continuation, readjustment, or cessation of the program (corrective action).

Product assessment, then, compares the final outcome with the stated objective and determines the degree of congruence.

POST-TEST 5–4

Define the three elements of product assessment.

FOCUS OF CONTROL SYSTEMS

Control is exercised over the money, manpower, and work of the health care institution. Control mechanisms for these resources comprise both structural and behavioral processes and include the budget, employee classification, training, evaluation, work review procedures, and peer pressure.

Monetary Control

A budget is prepared on the basis of anticipated income and proposed expenditures of resources over a given period of time. The budget provides a plan for resource allocation to operate the institution or department and to aid the manager in attaining institutional and departmental goals. A carefully prepared budget provides the manager with a tool to measure and compare actual results with a financial plan on a periodic basis. Budgetary plans generally include an overall financial plan for the organization as a whole and many sub-budgets for the various divisions and departments of the institution. The overall budget becomes the principal concern of the top administrator and the board of trustees, whereas the manager of a department becomes involved with his own departmental budget. The term *budgetary control* refers to the use of budgets to monitor the operations of a department so that they will be in conformity with the goals and standards articulated in the budget.

Using the control process model, budgets develop after the needs, goals, strategies, and plans for the institution have been defined. In other words, the budget offers a precise statement of resource allocation plans for specified programs for a future period.

During the process assessment phase, the financial estimates for each department provide inputs into an overall institutional program. For example, the cost of the housekeeping orientation program discussed earlier becomes part of the total training budget for the institution. Also during the process assessment phase, feedback reports go to the department heads to inform them of how their operation conforms to projected revenue and expense. Corrective action is taken when major discrepancies occur between the projected and actual figures.

At the end of the budget period, a determination of the feasibility of the current budget provides a base for the following year's financial planning. Was it realistic in terms of monetary obligations? Should it be changed? If so, in what areas? This information is recycled into a new financial program.

The departmental manager can use the budget as an effective control over the financial resources of his department if he coordinates the planning of programs with allocation of financial resources for these programs.

Budgeting improves planning by stimulating one to think about the future and leads to greater specificity in long- and short-range forecasting, since resources have to be allocated to each program in a comprehensive way.

The departmental manager should work with the financial officer of the institution in the preparation of the departmental budget. Prior to this, however, he should meet with the employees in his department to determine whether new programs should be started, how they should be staffed, and a realistic budget for their implementation. Involvement of the departmental staff also motivates the employees to stay within the defined budget, since they will have had a say in its development.

Budgeting reports provide an assessment of the performance of the departmental manager by showing whether his projected and actual income and expense are congruent. This type of monitoring also has an impact on employee performance. If a subordinate knows that his supervisor watches budget results closely and that unfavorable results lead to a request for explanation, he will try to avoid having to make such an explanation by keeping performance up to the budget standard. When deviations do occur, he will try to institute corrective action before being called into conference. On the other hand, if a manager permits unfavorable results to slip by without comment, the subordinate will soon regard the budget as a set of figures not to be taken very seriously.

Finally, the budget is a control mechanism that helps the departmental manager to determine how well his objectives for a certain time period have been met. If he has stayed within his budget, the objectives of the program were realistic and reflected sound program planning. On the other hand, if the year-end reports reveal excessive cost overruns, the planning and organizational activities of the department should be examined.

POST-TEST 5–5

Discuss the use of the budget as a mechanism for controlling money.

Manpower Control

A primary responsibility of managers is to insure that there are enough people with the proper qualifications to accomplish a particular job. Of equal importance, one should avoid employing more people than are necessary. Manpower control utilizes environmental, process, and product assessment in the activities of job classification, education, and training, performance evaluation, and professional peer review activities.

JOB CLASSIFICATION

The goal definition process of environmental assessment encompasses the total mission of the institution. From this flows the organization and classification of jobs needed to accomplish the institutional goals. The classification of jobs also determines an equitable pay structure for all employees, and high morale in employee groups comes from the knowledge that the pay they are receiving is comparable to that of other employees doing similar work.

In the health care system, the many different types of positions make a systematic arrangement of positions necessary. The characteristics of a job include the type of work, the level of difficulty and responsibility, and the qualifications required. Knowing the kind of work an employee does is essential in determining the job title. A data processer's work differs from that of a dietary aide. Thus the positions do not fall into the same group.

Work performed in health agencies ranges from the routine to the complex. The skills and judgment needed for a beginning maintenance worker differ from those demanded for a director of maintenance. In job classification, jobs are grouped by department and then by the level of work within the department. This system provides uniform treatment in arranging positions according to kinds and level of responsibility within the total organization. Within a department, the manager should know the level of difficulty and responsibility for each job and the qualifications required to perform it.

Position classification gives meaning to the policy of equal pay for equal work. It further promotes order by arrangement of work assignments. It assists in employee selection by facilitating comparison of an accurate position description with the qualifications of the employee. Furthermore, it provides guidelines for departmental performance appraisals and helps to identify training needs of the individual employee. The information generated by position classification is organized into a job description. Job descriptions are available for both the employee and supervisor and become a control factor in employee induction and evaluation.

EDUCATION PROGRAMS

Another aspect of manpower control occurs in the process assessment phase, when programs are staffed and in operation. Employees are organized and given authority to carry out certain segments of the work of a department. In order to insure that this work is of the highest quality, continuous education of the employee is essential. These programs deal with orientation, skill training, continuing education, and management development.

The orientation of new employees and newly transferred or promoted employees establishes a basis for mutual understanding of the supervisor's and employee's duties, responsibilities, authority, and relationships. A successful orientation program assists the employee in making a contribution to the institution and minimizes the possibility of errors and misunderstandings and the need for disciplinary action.

Orientation should be provided for all employees. Usually the orientation process consists of the broad orientation to the institution given by the personnel department, the departmental orientation given by the department head, and work-unit orientation given by the employees.

Skill Training. This type of educational program helps the employee to develop expertise in handling equipment and procedures necessary for carrying out his assigned work. If an employee is well trained in his job, there will be fewer equipment breakdowns, fewer patient complaints, fewer job errors, and a more productive work force.

Skill training can be done by the department head, as in the case of demonstrations about the use of laundry or maintenance equipment. This type of training can also be handled by the staff of the education department of a hospital or performed by an educational institution such as a vocational school. In the case of the nurse aide and the ward clerk, training programs are often conducted at an adult education center.

Continuing Education. These programs help the professional and nonprofessional staff to keep up with the trends and new procedures in their particular areas. Continuing education programs can be carried out within the institution or in conjunction with a professional organization or university.

Management Development. These programs are given to people within the organization who need the management skills of planning, organizing, directing, controlling, and coordinating. They can be offered as a consortium effort among many institutions or within the individual institution.

PERFORMANCE EVALUATION

The product assessment phase of control determines whether objectives were accomplished. Likewise, evaluation of the employee's performance determines whether he is accomplishing the work he was hired to perform.

Employee evaluation is a supervisory responsibility, which determines whether employee work performance meets established standards. The key to effective employee assessment rests with the supervisor.

One of the main tasks of the supervisor is to accomplish the particular work of his department through the efforts of others. His skill in motivating his work staff depends to a large extent on his ability to counsel, coach, and constructively criticize the work performance of his employees. The benefits achieved by a performance-evaluation system are proportional to the way in which the supervisor uses the mechanism for self-development of employees so that they will be aware of their strengths and weaknesses in job performance. If used as a punitive measure, the process can weaken productivity and motivation.

Performance appraisal should be a continuous process, not just a procedure performed at an anniversary date. Effective appraisal reveals to what extent actual performance meets standards, which aspects of performance need improvement, and to what extent the employee can develop further. Appraisal is based on a thorough knowledge of work standards and the employee's performance and the environmental conditions under which the work is performed. The evaluation should be written, signed by the employee and the supervisor, and kept in the employee's folder.

PEER REVIEW

People who take pride in their work perform well and expect their fellow workers to do the same. Countless examples of worker assistance and peer pressure to perform well are seen in the health care institution — the cook who encourages the person she is working with to add more seasoning so that the soup will be tasty, the nurse's aide who helps a younger worker to make a bed in the regal way so that the patients on their nursing team will be satisfied. Inferior performance reflects on everyone in a department regardless of who has actually done the work.

Peer review is especially noticeable among the professional workers in the hospital. The establishment of professional standards of performance has been a hallmark of a profession. This phenomenon is becoming increasingly important as the Professional Standards Review Organizations become operationalized and the stress on the auditing performance of health professionals grows in importance.

Managers should encourage the peer review process, since this is the most appropriate form of evaluation for professional workers. The departmental manager should insure that the worker groups have clearly defined standards of performance that can be used for reference and guidance.

POST-TEST 5–6

Describe four manpower control mechanisms.

Work Control

Monitoring the quality and flow of the work of a department represents another focus for the control process. Work control concerns itself primarily with maintaining the main functions of the department at a stable and efficient level. It also serves to point out causes of inefficiency and waste so they can be corrected. Such devices as work measurement and assignment of tasks are effective work supervising measures that can be used during the process and product assessment phases of control.

WORK MEASUREMENT

Managers must constantly look for ways to improve the flow and quality of work. Examination of existing work methods is usually the basis for improvement of the departmental work output. The first step in this process is to analyze the activity that consumes the most man-hours of the job, since improvement in this area will automatically influence the work of the total department. In analyzing work, the supervisor has to be aware of the flow of work, the methods used to do the work, and the number of tasks done in a procedure. Some of the questions that can be asked about each of these are as follows.

Work flow
Does the work come in at a steady rate?
Does work pile up before it can be processed?
Are there noticeable obstacles in the processing of work?
Is work being processed within a reasonable length of time?
Work methods
Are the methods appropriate to the work that is being performed?
Are the major steps in the work procedure clear?
Is each step in the procedure necessary?
At what point in the procedure is the most time expended?
Is the equipment appropriate for the work?
How many procedures have to be repeated?
Task analysis
Is a particular task essential to the total procedure?
Could one task be merged with another task?
Could the flow of tasks be altered?
Does the worker have skill in performing the task?
Such questions can be used to monitor work in progress. The information obtained from this type of analysis helps to define better work methods for the future and can be incorporated into a work procedure manual.

ASSIGNMENT OF WORK

Assignment of work is one of the activities of the process assessment phase of control. The supervisor chooses an individual with the necessary skills to perform a certain job and gives clear directions about the nature of the job to be performed. The supervisor can make a job assignment by giving oral or written instructions.

Oral instructions can be used effectively for minor work assignments, for clarifying written orders, and in emergencies. Oral instructions are often misunderstood when the manager speaks indistinctly or in a noisy area, when the orders are not organized in a logical sequence, and when the worker is inattentive.

Written instructions should be used when assigning work in another location, when the worker may be forgetful, when you wish to hold the workers responsible for the output, and when the task assignment is important and needs to be followed precisely. Written orders can be misunderstood when words with ambiguous meanings are used, when instructions are not arranged in sequence, and when the orders are too brief or incomplete.

Besides specific orders for each employee, a master work-assignment sheet for the shift or work period is a helpful control device. This master sheet insures that all the work will be assigned, and the supervisor can monitor the progress of the work attainment by periodically checking the documented assignment sheet.

Once the manager has assigned the work and has checked on its progress, he should have the employee report back on the completion of the job. This procedure reinforces accountability and gives the supervisor a chance to coordinate the total work effort, adjust deadlines, pinpoint trouble spots, and compliment the worker when he has done a good job.

POST-TEST 5–7

1. Define two mechanisms for monitoring work flow.
2. Analyze the organization of work in your area or department to see if it could be altered for greater efficiency and quality of output.

ELEMENTS OF A CONTROL SYSTEM

Before a management control system can be operative, four elements must be present. These are:
1. Organized planning process.
2. Development of organizational control tools.

3. Development of a coordinated information system.
4. Use of evaluation as a continuous process.

Organized Planning Process

Planning and control are companion management functions. Planning defines what *should* take place; control documents what *did* take place. If clear goals and objectives with acceptable performance criteria are written into the plans, the task of evaluation and control is much easier. Information used to monitor the progress of programs and to determine whether objectives have been met can be used in determining new needs, problems, and opportunities for future plans.

Development of Organizational Control Tools

The mechanisms for carrying out plans and programs are also important in implementing control systems. These organizational factors are a clear delineation of the total work of the institution, development of policies and procedures, delegation of authority and responsibility, delineation of span of control of managers, adequate communication channels, and standards of performance for every department of the hospital. These management practices clarify the institutional mission and the mechanisms for monitoring and achieving the mission.

Coordinated Information System

In order to define standards, pinpoint the exceptions, monitor the multiple operations of the organization, develop adequate reporting systems, and have the information needed for assessing new needs and problems in the environment, a coordinated information system is needed. This system is usually computer-based and provides an integrated data flow for all the decision-making activities in the institution.

Continual Evaluation

Evaluation is an ongoing process of determining the type of information that is needed for decision making. Evaluation formulation is needed to adequately recognize needs and formulate objectives. It is also needed while programs are being implemented, to see whether there are any obstacles to the program. Finally, a product evaluation is needed to determine whether a plan has adequately met its goals and objectives. This information is used to change, stop, or recycle a program, and the cycle begins again.

POST-TEST 5–8

What is necessary to implement a control system within your area of responsibility?

SUMMARY

A management control system is necessary to determine whether the goals of the organization are being met according to specified standards. The control function encompasses environmental, process, and product assessment. It is used in relation to the financial, manpower, and work processes of the organization. Effective control is dependent on an organized planning process, a coordinated information system, and continual evaluation.

RECAP EXERCISE 5

Mr. Jackson, the administrator of the hospital, has just informed you that the board of trustees has approved plans to begin a home care program. The activity will be based in the outpatient department and be supervised by yourself and the director of outpatient services. You will have a nurse, a social worker, two nurse aides, and a part-time physical therapist on the staff and will use the other resources and staff of the outpatient department when necessary.

Mr. Jackson would like the program to begin as soon as possible, but because it is an experimental program, he would like it monitored closely.

1. Define the steps you would go through in setting up control points for this program.

2. Who would you involve in this process?

REFERENCES

1. American Hospital Association: *Budgeting Procedures for Hospitals.* Chicago, American Hospital Association, 1971.
2. Anthony, R. N.: *Planning and Control Systems: A Framework for Analysis.* Boston, Division of Research, Harvard Business School, 1965.
3. Berman, Howard, Jr., and Weeks, Lewis E.: *Financial Management of Hospitals,* 2nd ed. Ann Arbor, Health Administration Press, 1974.
4. Eilor, Samuel: *Management Control.* New York, John Wiley & Sons, Inc., 1971.
5. Harris, Douglas H., and Chaney, Frederick B.: *Human Factors in Quality Assurance.* New York, John Wiley & Sons, Inc., 1969.

6. Hay, L.: *Budgeting and Cost Analyses for Hospital Management.* Bloomington, Ind., University Publications, 1958.
7. Mackenzie, R. Alex: *The Time Trap: Managing Your Way Out.* New York, AMACOM, American Management Association, 1972.
8. Miver, J. B., and Brewer, J. T.: The management of ineffective performance. In M. Dunnette (ed.): *Handbook of Industrial and Organizational Psychology.* Chicago, Rand-McNally, 1973.
9. Newport, M. Gene: *The Tools of Managing: Functions, Techniques and Skills.* Reading, Mass., Addison-Wesley Publishing Co., 1972.
10. Suaer, J.: Involvement of all managerial levels important to successful budgeting. *Hosp. Top. 47:*33, 1969.
11. Stufflebeam, Daniel L.: *Educational Evaluation and Decision Making.* Itasca, Ill., F. E. Peacock Publishers, Inc., 1971.
12. Tannebaum, A. S.: *Control in Organizations.* New York, McGraw-Hill Book Co., 1968.
13. Wildavsky, Aaron P.: *The Politics of the Budgetary Process.* Boston, Little, Brown and Co., 1964.
14. Griffith, John R.: Hancock, Walton M., and Munson, Fred C. (eds.): *Cost Control in Hospitals.* Ann Arbor, Health Administration Press, 1976.

Selected Readings

INTRODUCTION

Systems within organizations and between organizations in society are complex. To keep pace with the complexity of relationships, a new discipline, management, has matured to deal with the problems of bringing together large and diverse groups of people to work toward some common goals and for mutually rewarding purposes. Planning, organizing, and decision making are some of the common interrelated approaches to dealing with organizational problems. One of the most widely accepted approaches in dealing with complexity in organizations is management by objectives. Peter Drucker is a leading thinker and writer on this subject.

Curtis McLaughlin, working within a similar framework, deals with some of the control techniques available to the perceptive manager, which can be used within the overall management-by-objectives framework. Effective communication is the basis for working together, and Drucker believes that this will also occur best within a framework of management by objectives. McLaughlin stresses the need for planning and specific consideration of cost and performance in a formal management-by-objective approach in order to control results and evaluate performance. The conceptual chapters in this book stress this fundamental approach.

McLaughlin stresses the long-range strategic planning process. Limited resources require consideration of trade offs between what we want individually and what the organization can do best and can afford. He correctly points out that all of the members of the institution want to know what their "piece of the action" will be and what will happen to the programs that they consider important. Therefore, involvement in the process of decision making is important. One major way to insure that communication and agreement occur is to have each program level manager participate in setting his own targets and then participate in a process of questioning the assumptions of each element of the program. Assumptions are often neglected elements of major and minor programs. One of the longest debated assumptions is the notion that high cost and high quality tend to go together. Research in this area suggests that definitive controls can bring higher quality and lower cost. Planning and controlling of each element in the organization's work can pay off in producing better quality and improved cost performance; hence the strong recommendation of McLaughlin to check assumptions carefully.

Communication between people in organizations presents one of the most challenging problems facing managers in organizations. Drucker, in his book *Management: Tasks, Responsibilities, Practices*, gets at the heart of this problem in the framework of a management-by-objectives philosophy. He notes that the fundamental problems of communication occur

67

when the sender of information is unable to relate to the concepts, values, beliefs, and expectations of the person with whom he is communicating. One must know what it is that the receiver wishes, can accept, and needs to accomplish. In order to communicate, it is necessary to understand the motivations, values, and purpose of the person to whom one must relate. For these reasons Drucker feels that "downward communication" is doomed to failure unless one can first relate to what subordinates want to know and do, what they are interested in, and what they are ready to receive. His suggestion is that management by objectives, an underlying assumption expressed in the chapters on conceptual skills, can motivate each level of management within the organization to spell out what they want to do. The manager must help subordinates to understand constraints at different levels of the system and work with each employee to find an acceptable compromise that will be effective for the organization and its mission and the needs and goals of the individual. Effective communication can occur and performance can be improved within such a system of management.

Exercises

1. List three specific reasons why communication about cost controls from the administrator of your organization might face a lack of response from different persons within the organization. *(Hint:* The professional who views quality of care as a prime directive in his or her work might not value this type of consideration or at least not until what they feel they must and can do has been given full consideration.)

2. Your department has received a memo from the administration requesting that no personal calls be made on the organization's phones.
   a. What are some of the possible problems and needs that employees might express before any final decision about the use of organizational telephones for personal business can be resolved?
   b. Suggest a plan for getting subordinates to work out an effective performance goal to insure that personal communications are handled in the least costly fashion. Find out what others feel is necessary and ask for alternative ways of dealing with the problem. Consider whether there is a more effective way of dealing with the problem than an edict to stop using the telephones for personal business during working hours.

3. Take one of your own pet programs and use the assumption-testing approach suggested by McLaughlin to question each element of the program and see if you can find ways to change, modify, or even abandon the programs without lowering quality, abandoning a program of value, or raising cost.

Strategic Planning and Control in Small Health Organizations

CURTIS P. MCLAUGHLIN

Strategic or long-range planning is vitally important to the manager of the small health organization, but it is difficult for him to accept it as a practical process. Resources are limited, especially his time and energy as senior administrator-professional. His ability to influence the environment significantly is improbable; he has scant resources to apply to the projection and preparation for a future which is subject to rapid changes, even when it is limited to a three- to five-year horizon. The likelihood of a significant payoff often seems low. Yet every health manager knows that he is likely to end up in serious difficulties if the organization is merely swept along like a cork on a tide of external events. What is needed is a simple, relevant and low-cost planning approach. So the critical questions become "What do I need?" and "Where do I start, given my limited resources?". Where I stop expending those resources will depend on how valuable the experience ahead looks to me. Let's start with the latter question first.

ENTRÉE VIA BUDGET

The health manager knows that he needs all the help he can afford. Finding an efficient starting place, therefore, increases what the organization can afford; and cost can be reduced significantly by piggybacking the planning on necessary operating procedures.

Everyone has to deal with financial statements and to present budgets. At the very least these have to be developed to meet the requests of external organizations like banks, funding agencies, planning agencies, and boards of directors. While they are often based on uninteresting historical figures, they still can be the basic starting

Health Care Management Review 1:45–53, Winter, 1976.

point for a planning process. The information is usually current, available, consistent and reliable.

Since many health organizations have a well-developed budgeting and control procedure, the budgeting-control area may be the least-cost place to enter into the planning process. From there one can consider embellishing and reality-testing the plan in terms of the related choice areas: mix of services, personnel, pricing policies and cost controls, funding mix, marketing plans, and organizational structure. Remember, however, that budget constraints do not set policies with respect to these related choices. The budget process is merely an entry into the iterative, cyclical process of planning. Tradeoffs are made continuously between choice areas until an acceptable strategy and plan of action emerges for the organization's future.

PLANNING AND CONTROL SYSTEMS

In 1965 R. N. Anthony offered a useful and simple way of classifying some basic processes within organizations.[1] While his work was initially applied to industry, it has since been expanded to cover non-profit organizations.[2] He cited three processes for the internal organization: strategic planning, managerial control and operational control. These are separate and distinct from information processing and from more externally oriented financial accounting. According to Anthony,

- **Strategic planning** is the process of deciding on objectives of the organization, on changes in these objectives, on the resources used to attain these objectives, and on the policies that are to govern the acquisition, use and disposition of these resources.

- **Managerial control** is the process by which managers assure that resources are obtained and used effectively and efficiently toward the organization's objectives.

- **Operational control** is the process of assuring that specific tasks are carried out effectively and efficiently.

Table 1 lists the kinds of elements that seem necessary for the planning and control system of a health organization. All of these activities are necessary, even when the product is highly intangible and the organization is a nonprofit one. The word "marketing" may evoke concepts that conflict with your professional and personal values, but the fact remains that marketing is especially important in service organizations;[3, 4] and in public service organizations "he who pays the piper calls the tune." This implies that there are at least three constituencies to be marketed to—Pipers (professionals), Payors, and Dancers (clients). There may, in fact, be many more than three publics to be marketed to in the typical health program.[5]

STRATEGIC PLANNING

We are all familiar with the fact that form and quality of future revenue for health organizations is uncertain. For the nonprofit health organizations that do not provide direct care services to paying clients, it is highly uncertain. If the organization performs research or services for Federal, state or local governments or is reimbursed through their agencies, it is subject to all the whims of the appropriations process. In other cases there is dependence upon uncertain demand for services in the planning period or upon an annual fund-raising campaign.

But this is no excuse for avoiding a long-range budget or long-range funding projections—which may or may not be distinct from funding objectives. Only with such figures in view can the manager identify the need for changes in strategies with respect to growth, per-

Table 1   Elements of a Budget and Control System for a Small Health Organization

---

STRATEGIC PLANNING
Long-range strategic budget
   By objective or program
   By function or item classification
Long-range funding projections
   By objective or program
   By function or item classification
   By potential sourcing
   By flexibility category or degree or discretionality
Evaluation reporting and organizational structure
Marketing strategy

MANAGERIAL CONTROL
Cash flow projections (by month for six to twelve months)
Budget
   By objective or program
   By function or item classification
   By source or grant
Budget control—cumulative expenditures and commitments
     versus projected rates of activity
   By objective or program
   By function or item classification
   By source or grant
Activity vs. objectives comparison
Manpower budgets and training plans
Marketing plans

OPERATIONAL CONTROL
Cash and bank account control and reporting
Receivables and payable control and reporting
Trial balance, audit, preaudit and accrual activities
Property control
Grants accounting and reporting
Position control
Activity reporting

---

sonnel, funds acquisition, investment, mix and scope of services and activities, and marketing strategy.

Table 1 implies both a budget by program and one by function or items. There has been long and heated debate about the merits of program budgeting versus line-item budgeting. There is no doubt that the program budget is more important in long-range planning. Health organizations run programs; basically, they are to be judged by the success of those programs. Line-item budgets carry a very limiting underlying assumption. They fix the factors of production that the manager is supposed to be selecting and combining to produce program results. They imply an assumption that the manager is incompetent to carry out one of a manager's most important tasks—allocating resources to make a program effective.

But sooner rather than later the manager of a health organization will translate the program budget into line items for two reasons: Funding agencies and the program manager's supervisors will want to look at specific items, especially professional and nonprofessional personnel, travel and supplies; and the managers of care delivery and support subunits will want to know what specifically they will have to work with and be responsible for.

This breakdown by function or item classification is especially necessary if the manager chooses to involve subunit managers in planning. Even though the head of a health organization thinks entirely in program terms, each successive level down the hierarchy that participates in the process must think less in program terms and more in terms of the specifics that he or she deals with. Regardless of how many programs are involved, the pharmacist will want to see a drug budget, the director of nursing the funds available from all sources for paying nurses, and the motor pool manager the transportation funds allocated there. And the manager who does not encourage subunit managers to participate in the planning process may lose both technical skills and future commitment on the part of the staff.

FOUR LONG-RANGE FUNDING PROJECTIONS

In organizations with multiple programs and multiple funding sources it is useful to prepare four funding projections. The first two of these, as shown in Table 1, correspond directly to the two strategic budgets. The third is a projection by potential sources of funds which may or may not bear a close relationship to the program budget. Preparing this projection is not time consuming, and it has the advantage of highlighting quickly the major needs or opportunities for strategic changes in program direction, and for marketing the organization to funding sources.

The fourth category of breakdown is added to focus attention on the need to acquire discretionary funding rather than funding which is restricted to specific line items or program activities. It is a rare health organization which receives exactly the mix of fundings, and permissions to spend them, that meets its total needs. This is especially true of the seed money necessary for program development, staff development, travel, entertainment, reference materials, and so forth. Yet the manager must recognize that some funds for such purposes may be critical to the survival of the organization. In some cases it is customary to acquire funding for work that already is partially completed in order to make funds available to develop the next contract. This play requires a constant feed-forward of work and money. The endowment income on general purpose donations to a local organization is often its only discretionary resource. Without the requisite amount of flexible resources it is very difficult to have a holistic, coherent strategy and maintain the appropriate set of people and programs.

Even a relatively homogenous, small and profit-oriented organization like a group medical or dental practice needs to think in terms of flexible funding for staff development, equipment improvements, pet projects, etc. If all the new income is passed through to the partners or associates, there is little motivation to make the practice more coherent and effective. If the practice is highly solvent, it is wise to build up a kitty for practice flexibility and improvement, if for no better reason than to force the partners to discuss whether or not there are group goals as well as individual goals and to provide an impetus for striving toward them.

THE PLANNING CYCLE

Having prepared budget and funds projection, the small health organization is likely to identify gaps in funding sources, programs, or both. One relatively easy way to visualize this is in a chart like Figure 1.

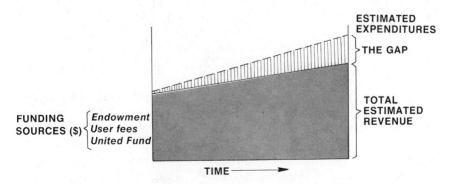

Figure 1 Identifying the Gap.

Then it becomes necessary to look at the assumptions leading to these conditions, with or without a gap. This can be and usually is approached from two sides. One is to examine the alternatives for solutions to observed problems in meeting the objectives. The second is to test out the sequence of assumptions used with respect to needs, costs, prices, manpower, program acceptability, social attitudes, professional attitudes, and interorganizational relationships.

Peter Drucker[6] has outlined quite succinctly planning steps for a service organization. They are:

1. Define what is the "business" and what it should be. This should be an open consideration of alternative needs to be met and reasons for being.

2. Derive from this clear set of goals and objectives.

3. Think through the priorities for concentrating efforts on targets, standards of performance for these targets, setting deadlines and getting down to work.

4. Define measures of performance.

5. Provide for review (audit) of the outcomes to see which are acceptable and where effort should be directed toward change. This should include a mechanism for "sloughing off" unproductive activities. Macleod's article entitled "Program Budgeting Works in Nonprofit Institutions" is a good illustration of how small, unsophisticated health organization was able to go through this process and even ended up sloughing off some services that its constituency was unwilling to support.[7]

The health system manager likes to think of himself or herself as a person who deals primarily with the facts. Yet the process of management really is based on a large number of assumptions. The trick is to identify those to which the management plan is most sensitive and conduct experiments with that subset which you are least sure of *and,* if proved untrue, would lead to significant changes in effectiveness.

Examples of critical assumptions in health are:

● People will not accept primary care from nonphysicians.
● Medical care usage is not sensitive to prices.
● Group therapy is cheaper than individual therapy.
● HMOs are the way to cut health care costs.
● Nurse practitioners will work out well in rural settings.
● Building a new medical school at our end of the state will mean more available primary care.
● Government funding and reimbursement principles will remain consistent.
● People will accept primary care from nonphysicians.

The alert manager will set up situations that probe in the direction of testing such assumptions. Controlled experiments are often out of the question, even in large organizations. The pressure of day-to-day demands and the fact that there are one-of-a-kind facilities preclude them. But it is possible to build up a set of data from natural events and from probing experiences to see whether or not a change might make sense over the long haul.

EXIT ANYWHERE

Assumption tests could affect all stages of the planning cycle as illustrated in Figure 2. The sequence around the large loop in Figure 2 is not a fixed one. Rationales can be made for numerous changes in sequencing, but the purpose of the diagram here is to lay out these activities for the manager of the small health organization, not to provide *the* sequence.

The most unusual box is labeled "coherency check" and is linked to the flexible funds projection. It is there to emphasize the necessity for the health manager to step back and see whether or not all the people and activities around his shop add up to something that makes sense, is balanced and coherent, and feels right.

On the microcosmic level we have the same problems with task analysis for employees. We can define tasks and the skills necessary to perform specific health procedures. Yet we have no assurances that at a given time and place these tasks and skills can be combined into a meaningful job and a meaningful role. Similarly, a community mental health organization may provide the five mandated services and sev-

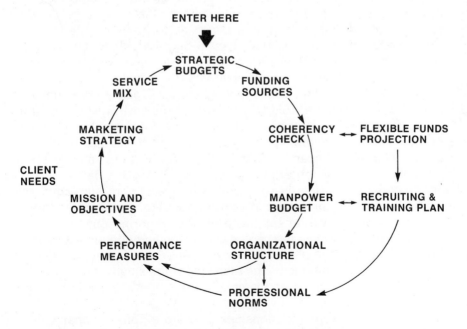

Figure 2   The long-range planning process.

eral others and still not make much sense as an entity. It is an important duty of the leadership to see that all the pieces (programs) fit together and that the employees understand this.

The sequence in Figure 2 is most likely to be challenged on the grounds of "which comes first, the chicken or the egg." The order is derived from the entry point and the exit points that the manager of a small health organization might well choose. Every manager ought to be willing to go around the loop periodically thinking in broad conceptual terms. After that he has to make careful choices about how much time and resources should go into the detailed phases of planning, then consider whether or not to go into an even more detailed system like "management-by-objectives" with written plans, mission statements, performance targets, client satisfaction and need surveys, employee attitude surveys, and so forth.

The outcome of a very modest investment might be as simple, but powerful, as the idea that we need to fund and add an additional nursing auxiliary in late 1976; and we need to keep an eye on how new Social Security programs affect our ability to bill for specific services and our willingness to purchase specific diagnostic equipment.

WHERE DOES THE ENVIRONMENT FIT IN?

Much has been said about the details of the strategic planning process, but Anthony and Herzlinger point out that it is "largely unsystematic and informal." Decisions are made at irregular intervals and the information required usually has to be developed specifically for the issues involved.[8] They also cite the well-known fact that this involves a continual watch on the environment.

Figure 2, therefore, does not specifically place environmental inputs into that picture. This is because a single environmental change could impinge on several boxes at once. Take, for example, the impact of unionization on the operations of a developmental disabilities center. The initial impact is likely to be upon wage rates and appear immediately in the long-range budgeting area. But bargaining on "non-economic" issues is very likely to involve work standards and methods which in turn affect manpower budgets, recruiting and training plans, conflict with or support professional norms, change marketing strategy and service mix, and even affect accreditation aspirations. Some of these will impact choice areas sequentially, while others will be impinged upon uniquely. The manager of the small institution must accept that the impacts of major environmental shifts can be quite varied and pervasive.

Interorganizational relationships also are a natural consideration for the health manager, but are presumably of more interest to larger organizations. Space considerations preclude dealing with this topic here, except to say that Kenneth Benson's observations on domain consensus and ideological consensus are especially relevant to health organizations.[9]

WHERE DOES EVALUATION FIT IN?

Evaluation inputs should be a part of this planning process. In the typical service program, the evaluation effort should be aimed at setting objectives and selectively allocating resources that will improve the internal operation and the outputs delivered to and impacting on the public. Evaluation efforts which are not keyed to internal information needs fall at best into the financial reporting category, or are idle exercise or specialized professional skills.

MANAGERIAL CONTROL

The small health organization may be able to do strategy planning, but its efforts will be worth a great deal more in the long run if they are linked to the implementation stages of managerial control and operational control. Although I am focusing here on the strategic planning process, it seems important to deal with managerial and operational control in conjunction with strategic planning.

Cash flow projections are critical to the survival of the organization. Even an organization making a profit can fail if it lacks the cash to meet its payroll or to satisfy the least patient of its creditors. This is also the case with a nonprofit organization. The amount of effort devoted to this activity will fluctuate depending on the variability or seasonability of cash flows. Cash flow projection is a shorter-range counterpart to funding projections.

Budgeting is something that all organizations quickly learn to live with. In order to end up without a loss each individual must have a specific commitment to expend only a specific amount of resources and then stick to that commitment. Here, as in the case of strategic planning, it probably will prove necessary to live with three sets of budgetary breakdowns—four if the concern for flexibility of funding is carried through at this level of control.

The budget process, if carefully administered, is a major opportunity for the manager to motivate the behavior of personnel in individual subunits of the organization. If the budget is imposed from the "top down" then there is often little felt obligation to establish the ends of the subunits within that constraint. Either the subunit will try to overspend to meet its goals, or feel justified in not meeting those goals because inadequate resources are provided. The only way to avoid this impasse is to have the subunit manager participate in a "button-up" development of the budget. This does not imply that there may not be drastic cuts from the initial requests, but these should be arrived at in conjunction with the setting of operational objectives. Only then can there be a mutual contract between the employees and the management to perform set tasks with allowed resources. A good description of this negotiation process can be found in Wildavsky's *The Politics of the Budgetary Process.*[10]

While budgets are a useful projection and negotiation device, the real day-to-day planning and control tool lies within the process of comparing the expenditures and encumbrances with the amounts that the budget planning process indicated should have been consumed at any given point in time. Table 2 gives a statement of financial condition for a crippled children's program and illustrates the utility of such a tool. It gives the total amount budgeted for the program, the amount expended and the balance remaining by item classification. An additional column represents moneys which have not been paid out, but for which there already is a commitment to expend them. This, subtracted from the cash balance, indicates how much is available for future decision-making. For example, the program budget period is only half complete, but the staff has already been hired and no more salary money can be committed. The item for travel is already due to be overspent. Assuming that a constant expenditure rate was planned, the program manager might question responsible subunit heads about the low rate of expenditure for foster home care, appliances, public health nurses, and health education. One might also wonder whether any plans had been made for staff training. If the rate of expenditure was not planned to be constant, then an additional column should have been added to show projected expenditures and encumbrances for the same cumulative period. Sometimes percentage columns are also provided.

It is important that the accounting system be set up on an accrual basis rather than a cash basis to give comparative information. If expenditures are compared monthly and some employees are paid weekly, portions of the pay periods which are in either the preceding or following periods should be added into the period results. Certain charges which are paid only yearly, like insurance, could also be spread out over the year, especially if such analyses are used to estimate appropriate service charges.

Also at the managerial control level, there has to be an equivalent of evaluation as it was discussed at the strategic planning level. This means keeping track of objectives or service statistics of the program and comparing them with resource inputs during the period. Such comparisons are a useful indicator of whether or not the current process seems to be effective and efficient. Some analysts equate evaluation primarily with outcome or benefit measurement. But, while that

Table 2   Budget Report—As of Halfway Mark in Budget Period—Crippled Children's Program*

BUDGET ITEM	AMOUNT BUDGETED	BUDGET AMOUNT EXPENDED	UNEXPENDED AMOUNT	AMOUNT COMMITTED	UNCOMMITTED BALANCE AVAILABLE
Salaries of Staff	$ 40,000	$17,500	$22,500	$22,500	$ 0
Physicians' Fees	20,000	11,000	9,000	2,000	7,000
Clinic Physicians' Fees	10,000	3,500	6,500	1,500	5,000
Hospitalization	35,000	18,000	17,000	2,500	14,500
Convalescent and Foster Home Care	4,000	500	3,500	250	3,250
Appliances	5,000	1,000	4,000	0	4,000
Drugs and Biologicals	500	200	300	0	300
X-ray and Laboratory Work	2,500	1,000	1,500	500	1,000
Staff Training	3,000	0	3,000	0	3,000
Travel	2,500	2,500	0	300	(300)
Equipment and Supplies	1,000	800	200	100	100
Publications, etc.	500	0	500	250	250
CC Subtotal	124,000	56,000	68,000	29,900	38,100
Administrative Offices	5,000	4,500	500	500	0
Health Education	4,000	500	3,500	500	3,000
Vital Statistics	2,000	1,700	300	50	250
Local Health Offices	5,000	1,000	4,000	1,000	3,000
Public Health Nursing	10,000	1,000	9,000	0	9,000
Supporting Subtotal	26,000	8,700	17,300	2,050	15,250
Total	150,000	64,700	85,300	31,950	53,350

*Adapted from data in How to use financial data as a basic program planning tool. In *Am. J. Public Health* 44:149–157, February, 1954.

is a very important type of information to the program manager, in social programs that measure comes only after considerable time has elapsed and may or may not be traceable to program activities. The manager, in the meantime, must modify program planning assumptions constantly and adjust the input and process stages in order to continue to improve operations. It is too costly to wait for the outcome evaluation before refining the process. The same holds in the manpower and marketing areas.

OPERATIONAL CONTROL

There are numerous things to keep track of in the health organization, especially when there are multiple sources of funds and many publics to be responsible to. The lack of authorization to incur openly either a profit or a loss means that controls, especially those over hiring and spending, must aim for particularly tight targets. Hiring controls are especially important since most health organizations provide intangible products and are labor intensive. Cash and bank account control, and control over payables and receivables, are common to any organization. Similarly the accounting activity of accruals, audits and trial balances is similar to that of a manufacturing organization. There is, however, especially in government organizations, the preaudit phase which requires that the expender have a budget officer review the contract to make sure that funds are still available within the constraints of budgets, and to assess whether purchasing (bidding), personnel, and other requirements have been met. Since public property and government employees and money may be involved, one may have to add property control, position control, and grants accounting and reporting to the control system.

Then the management must add activity reporting as the basis for process decision and for evaluation in support of grants reporting, managerial control, and strategic planning.

NONE TOO SMALL

It is important that the manager of a small health organization become familiar with the total processes of strategic planning and control even if he or she does not get into it in great depth or detail. It can have considerable impact on the effectiveness—even the survival—of the organization. It is not as complicated as budget analysts and program planning experts might like you to believe. It is not something to leave to accountants, agencies or staff analysts. It is worth understanding and considering actively, regardless of your scale of operations.

REFERENCES

1. Anthony, R. N.: *Planning and Control Systems: A Framework for Analysis.* Boston, Mass., Division of Research, Harvard University Graduate School of Business Administration, 1965.
2. Anthony, R. N., and Herzlinger, R. E.: *Management Control in Nonprofit Organizations.* Homewood, Ill., Richard D. Irwin, Inc., 1975.
3. Rathmell, J. M.: *Marketing in the Service Sector.* Cambridge, Mass., Winthrop Publishers, Inc., 1974.
4. Shapiro, B. P.: "Marketing for Nonprofit Organizations," *Harvard Business Review*, September-October, 1973, pp. 123–132.
5. Kotler, P.: *Marketing for Nonprofit Organizations.* Englewood Clifs, N. J., Prentice-Hall, Inc., 1975.
6. Drucker, P. F.: *Management.* New York, Harper and Row, 1974. Chapters 12, 13, and 14.
7. Macleod, R. K.: "Program Budgeting Works in Nonprofit Institutions," *Harvard Business Review*, September-October, 1971, pp. 59–69.
8. Anthony and Herzlinger: *Management Control in Nonprofit Organizations*, p. 28.
9. Benson, J. K.: "The Interorganizational Network as a Political Economy," *Administrative Science Quarterly*, 20, June 1975, pp. 229–249.
10. Wildavsky, A.: *The Politics of the Budgetary Process.* Boston, Mass., Little, Brown and Co., 1964. Chapter 1.

Managerial Communications

PETER F. DRUCKER

More Talk; and Less Communication—What We Have Learned—The Fundamentals—Communication Is Perception—Communication Is Expectation—Communication Makes Demands—Communication and Information Are Different—Information Presupposes Communication—Why Downward Communications Cannot Work—The Limitations of "Listening"—The Demands of the Information Explosion—What Can Managers Do?—Management by Objectives, Performance Appraisal and Management Letter as Communications Tools—Communications, the Mode of Organization

We have more attempts at communications today, that is, more attempts to talk to others, and a surfeit of communications media, unimaginable to the men who, around the time of World War I, started to work on the problems of communicating in organizations. Communications in management has become a central concern to students and practitioners in all institutions—business, the military, public administration, hospital, university, and research. In no other area have intelligent men and women worked harder or with greater dedication than psychologists, human relations experts, managers, and management students have worked on improving communications in our major institutions.

Yet communications has proven as elusive as the Unicorn. The noise level has gone up so fast that no one can really listen any more to all that babble about communications. But there is clearly less and less communicating. The communications gap within institutions and between groups in society has been widening steadily—to the point where it threatens to become an unbridgeable gulf of total misunderstanding.

In the meantime, there is an information explosion. Every professional and every executive—in fact, everyone except the deaf-mute—suddenly has access to data in inexhaustible abundance. All of us feel—and overeat—very much like the little boy who has been left alone in the candy store. But what has to be done to make this cornucopia of data redound to information, let alone to knowledge? We get a great many answers. But the one thing clear so far is that no one really has an answer. Despite information theory and data processing, no one yet has actually seen, let alone used, an "information system," or a "data base." The one thing we do know, though, is that the abundance of information changes the communications problem and makes it both more urgent and even less tractable.

There is a tendency today to give up on communications. In psychology, for instance, the fashion today is the T-group with its sensitivity training. The avowed aim is not communications, but self-awareness. T-groups focus on the "I" and not on the "Thou." Ten or twenty years ago the rhetoric stressed "empathy"; now it stresses "doing one's thing." However needed self-knowledge may be, communication is needed at least as much (if indeed self-knowledge is possible without action on others, that is, without communications).

Despite the sorry state of communications in theory and practice, we have learned a good deal about information and communications. Most of it, though, has not come out of the work on communications to which we have devoted so much time and energy. It has been the by-product of work in a large number of seemingly unrelated fields, from learning theory to genetics and electronic engineering. We equally have a lot of experience—though mostly of failure—in a good many practical situations in all kinds of institutions. We may indeed never understand "communications." But "communications in organizations"—call it *managerial communications*—we do know something about by now.

We are, to be sure, still far away from mastery of communications, even in organizations. What knowledge we have about communications is scattered and, as a rule, not accessible, let alone in applicable form. But at least we increasingly know what does not work, and, sometimes, why it does not work. Indeed we can say bluntly that most of today's brave attempts at communication in organizations—whether business, labor unions, government agencies, or universities—is based on assumptions that have been proven to be invalid—and that, therefore, these efforts cannot have results. And perhaps we can even anticipate what might work.

WHAT WE HAVE LEARNED

We have learned, mostly through doing the wrong things, four fundamentals of communications.

1. Communication is perception.
2. Communication is expectation.
3. Communication makes demands.
4. Communication and information are different and indeed largely opposite—yet interdependent.

1. *Communication is perception.* An old riddle posed by the mystics of many religions—the Zen Buddhists, the Sufis of Islam, and the Rabbis of the Talmud—asks: "Is there a sound in the forest if a tree crashes down and no one is around to hear it?" We now know that the right answer to this is no. There are sound waves. But there is no sound unless someone perceives it. Sound is created by perception. Sound is communication.

This may seem trite; after all, the mystics of old already knew this, for they too always answered that there is no sound unless someone can hear it. Yet the implications of this rather trite statement are great indeed.

First, it means that it is the recipient who communicates. The so-called communicator, the person who emits the communication, does not communicate. He utters. Unless there is someone who hears, there is no communication. There is only noise. The communicator speaks or writes or sings—but he does not communicate. Indeed, he cannot communicate. He can only make it possible, or impossible, for a recipient—or rather, "percipient"—to perceive.

Perception, we know, is not logic. It is experience. This means, in the first place, that one always perceives a configuration. One cannot perceive single specifics. They are always part of a total picture. The "silent language,"* that is, the gestures, the tone of voice, the environment altogether, not to mention the cultural and social referents, cannot be dissociated from the spoken language. In fact, without them the spoken word has no meaning and cannot communicate.

It is not only that the same words, e.g., "I enjoyed meeting you," will be heard as having a wide variety of meanings. Whether they are heard as warmth or as icy cold, as endearment or as rejection depends on their setting in the "silent language," such as the tone of voice or the occasion. More important is that by itself, that is, without being part of the total configuration of occasion, value, "silent language,"

---

*As Edward T. Hall called it in the title of his pioneering work (Doubleday, 1959).

and so on, the phrase has no meaning at all. By itself it cannot make possible communication. It cannot be understood. Indeed it cannot be heard. To paraphrase an old proverb of the human-relations school: "One cannot communicate a word; the whole man always comes with it."

But we know about perception also that one can perceive only what one is capable of perceiving. Just as the human ear does not hear sounds above a certain pitch, so does human perception altogether not perceive what is beyond its range of perception. It may, of course, hear physically, or see visually, but it cannot accept it. It cannot become communication.

This is a fancy way of stating something the teachers of rhetoric have known for a very long time — though the practitioners of communications tend to forget it again and again.

In Plato's *Phaedo* which, among other things, is also the earliest extant treatise on rhetoric, Socrates points out that one has to talk to people in terms of their own experience, that is, that one has to use carpenters' metaphors when talking to carpenters, and so on. One can communicate only in the recipient's language or in his terms. And the terms have to be experience-based. It, therefore, does very little good to try to explain terms to people. They will not be able to receive them if they are not terms of their own experience. They simply exceed their perception capacity.

The connection between experience, perception, and concept formation — that is, cognition — is, we now know, infinitely subtler and richer than any earlier philosopher imagined. But one fact is proven and comes out strongly in the most disparate work, e.g., that of Piaget (in Switzerland), that of B. F. Skinner, and that of Jerome Bruner (both at Harvard). Percept and concept in the learner, whether child or adult, are not separate. We cannot perceive unless we also conceive. But we also cannot form concepts unless we can perceive. To communicate a concept is impossible unless the recipient can perceive it, that is, unless it is within his perception.

There is a very old saying among writers: "Difficulties with a sentence mean confused thinking. It is not the sentence that needs straightening out, it is the thought behind it." In writing we attempt, first, to communicate with ourselves. An "unclear sentence" is one that exceeds our own capacity for perception. Working on the sentence, that is, working on what is normally called communications, cannot solve the problem. We have to work on our own concepts first to be able to understand what we are trying to say — and only then can we write the sentence.

In communicating, whatever the medium, the first question has to be "Is this communication within the recipient's range of perception? Can he receive it?"

The "range of perception" is, of course, physiological and largely (though not entirely) set by physical limitations of man's animal body. When we speak of communication, however, the most important limitations on perception are usually cultural and emotional rather than physical.

That fanatics are not being convinced by rational arguments, we have known for thousands of years. Now we are beginning to understand that it is not "argument" that is lacking. Fanatics do not have the ability to perceive a communication which goes beyond their range of emotions. First their emotions would have to be altered. In other words, no one is really "in touch with reality," If by that we mean that he has complete openness to evidence. The distinction between "sanity" and "paranoia" does not lie in the ability to perceive, but in the ability to learn, that is, in the ability to change one's emotions on the basis of experience.

That perception is conditioned by what we are capable of perceiving was realized forty years ago by the most quoted but probably least heeded of all students of organization, Mary Parker Follett (e.g., especially in her collected essays, *Dynamic Administration,* Harper's, 1941). Follett taught that a disagreement or a conflict is likely not to be about the answers, or indeed about anything ostensible. It is, in most cases, the result of incongruity in perceptions. What A sees so vividly, B does not see at all. And, therefore, what A argues, has no pertinence to B's concerns, and vice versa. Both, Follett argued, are likely to see reality. But each is likely to see a different aspect of it. The world, and not only the material world, is multidimensional. Yet one can see only one dimension at a time.

One rarely realizes that there could be other dimensions, and that something that is so obvious to us and so clearly validated by our emotional experience has other dimensions, a "back" and "sides," which are entirely different and which, therefore, lead to entirely different perceptions. The story I mentioned earlier about the blind men and the elephant in which each one, encountering this strange beast, feels one of the elephant's parts, his leg, his trunk, his hide, and reports an entirely different conclusion, and holds to it tenaciously, is simply a metaphor of the human condition. There is no possibility of communication until this is understood and until he who has felt the hide of the elephant goes over to him who has felt the leg and feels the leg himself. There is no possibility of communications, in other words, unless we first know what the recipient, the true communicator, can see and why.

2. *Communication is expectation.* We perceive, as a rule, what we expect to perceive. We see largely what we expect to see, and we hear largely what we expect to hear. That the unexpected may be resented is not the important thing—though most of the work on communications in business and government thinks it is. What is truly im-

portant is that the unexpected is usually not received at all. It is not seen or heard, but ignored. Or it is misunderstood, that is, mis-seen or mis-heard as the expected.

On this we now have a century or more of experimentation. The results are unambiguous. The human mind attempts to fit impressions and stimuli into a frame of expectations. It resists vigorously any attempts to make it "change its mind," that is, to perceive what it does not expect to perceive or not to perceive what it expects to perceive. It is, of course, possible to alert the human mind to the fact that what it perceives is contrary to its expectations. But this first requires that we understand what it expects to perceive. It then requires that there be an unmistakable signal — "this is different," that is, a shock which breaks continuity. A gradual change in which the mind is supposedly led by small, incremental steps to realize that what is perceived is not what it expects to perceive will not work. It will rather reinforce the expectations and will make it even more certain that what will be perceived is what the recipient expects to perceive.

Before we can communicate, we must, therefore, know what the recipient expects to see and hear. Only then can we know whether communication can utilize his expectations — and what they are — or whether there is need for the "shock of alienation," for an "awakening" that breaks through the recipient's expectations and forces him to realize that the unexpected is happening.

3. *Communication makes demands.* Many years ago psychologists stumbled on a strange phenomenon in their studies of memory, a phenomenon that, at first, upset all their hypotheses. In order to test memory, the psychologists compiled a list of words to be shown to their experimental subjects for varying times as a test of their retention capacity. As control, a list of nonsense words, mere jumbles of letters, was devised. Much to the surprise of these early experimenters almost a century ago or so, their subjects (mostly students, of course) showed totally uneven memory retention of individual words. More surprising, they showed amazingly high retention of the nonsense words. The explanation of the first phenomenon is fairly obvious. Words are not mere information. They do carry emotional charges. And, therefore words with unpleasant or threatening associations tend to be suppressed, words with pleasant associations retained. In fact, this selective retention by emotional association has since been used to construct tests for emotional disorders and for personality profiles.

The relatively high retention rate of nonsense words was a greater puzzle. It was expected that no one would really remember words that had no meaning at all. But it has become clear over the years that the memory for these words, though limited, exists precisely because these words have no meaning. For this reason, they make no demand. They are truly neutral. With respect to them, memory could be said to be truly "mechanical," showing neither emotional preference nor emotional rejection.

A similar phenomenon, known to every newspaper editor, is the amazingly high readership and retention of the "fillers," the little three- or five-line bits of irrelevant incidental information that are used to "balance" a page. Why should anybody want to read, let alone remember, that it first became fashionable to wear different-colored hose on each leg at the court of some long-forgotten duke? Or, when and where baking powder was first used? Yet there is no doubt that these little tidbits of irrelevancy are read and, above all, that they are remembered, far better than almost anything else in the daily paper except the screaming headlines of the catastrophes. The answer is that the fillers make no demands. It is their total irrelevancy that accounts for their being remembered.

Communication is always "propaganda." The emitter always wants "to get something across." Propaganda, we now know, is both a great deal more powerful than the rationalists with their belief in "open discussion" believe, and a great deal less powerful than the myth-makers of propaganda, e.g., Dr. Goebbels in the Nazi regime, believed and wanted us to believe. Indeed the danger of total propaganda is not that the propaganda will be believed. The danger is that nothing will be believed and that every communication becomes suspect. In the end, no communication is being received. Everything anyone says is considered a demand and is resisted, resented, and in effect not heard at all. The end results of total propaganda are not fanatics, but cynics—but this, of course, may be even greater and more dangerous corruption.

Communication, in other words, always makes demands. It always demands that the recipient become somebody, do something, believe something. It always appeals to motivation. If, in other words, communication fits in with the aspirations, the values, the purposes of the recipient, it is powerful. If it goes against his aspirations, his values, his motivations, it is likely not to be received at all or, at best, to be resisted. Of course, at its most powerful, communication brings about "conversion," that is, a change of personality, of values, beliefs, aspirations. But this is the rare, existential event, and one against which the basic psychological forces of every human being are strongly organized. Even the Lord, the Bible reports, first had to strike Saul blind before he could raise him up as Paul. Communications aiming at conversion demand surrender. By and large, therefore, there is no communication unless the message can key in to the recipient's own values, at least to some degree.

4. *Communication and information are different and indeed largely opposite—yet interdependent.* Where communication is perception, information is logic. As such, information is purely formal and

has no meaning. It is impersonal rather than interpersonal. The more it can be freed of the human component, that is, of such things as emotions and values, expectations and perceptions, the more valid and reliable does it become. Indeed it becomes increasingly informative.

All through history, the problem has been how to glean a little information out of communications, that is, out of relationships between people, based on perception. All through history, the problem has been to isolate the information content from an abundance of perception. Now, all of a sudden, we have the capacity to provide information—both because of the conceptual work of the logicians (especially the symbolic logic of Russell and Whitehead, which appeared in 1910), and because of the technical work on data processing and data storage, that is, especially because of the computer and its tremendous capacity to store, manipulate, and transmit data. Now, in other words, we have the opposite problem from the one mankind has always been struggling with. Now we have the problem of handling information per se, devoid of any communication content.

The requirements for effective information are the opposite of those for effective communication. Information is, for instance, always specific. We perceive a configuration in communications; but we convey specific individual data in the information process. Indeed, information is, above all, a principle of economy. The fewer data needed, the better the information. And an overload of information, that is, anything much beyond what is truly needed, leads to information blackout. It does not enrich, but impoverishes.

At the same time, information presupposes communication. Information is always encoded. To be received, let alone to be used, the code must be known and understood by the recipient. This requires prior agreement, that is, some communication. At the very least, the recipient has to know what the data pertain to. Are the figures on a piece of computer tape the height of mountaintops or the cash balances of Federal Reserve member banks? In either case, the recipient would have to know what mountains are or what banks are to get any information out of the data.

The prototype information system may well have been the peculiar language known as *Armee Deutsch* (Army German) which served as language of command in the Imperial Austrian Army prior to 1918. A polyglot army in which officers, noncommissioned officers, and men often had no language in common, it functioned remarkably well with fewer than two hundred specific words—"fire," for instance, or "at ease," each of which had only one totally unambiguous meaning. The meaning was always an action. And the words were learned in and through actions, i.e., in what behaviorists now call "operant conditioning." The tensions in the Austrian Army after many decades of nationalist turmoil were very great indeed. Social intercourse between members of different nationalities serving in the same unit became increasingly difficult, if not impossible. But to the very end, the information system functioned. It was completely formal; completely rigid; completely logical in that each word had only one possible meaning; and it rested on completely pre-established communication regarding the specific response to a certain set of sound waves. This example, however, shows also that the effectiveness of an information system depends on the willingness and ability to think through carefully what information is needed by whom for what purposes, and then on the systematic creation of communication among the various parties to the system as to the meaning of each specific input and output. The effectiveness, in other words, depends on the pre-establishment of communication.

Communication communicates the more levels of meaning it has and the less it lends itself to quantification.

Medieval esthetics held that a work of art communicates on a number of levels, at least three if not four: the literal; the metaphorical; the allegorical; and the symbolic. The work of art that most consciously converted this theory into artistic practice was Dante's *Divina Commedia.* If by "information" we mean something that can be quantified, then the *Divina Commedia* is without any information content whatever. But it is precisely the ambiguity, the multiplicity of levels on which this book can be read, from being a fairy tale to being a grand synthesis of metaphysics, that makes it the overpowering work of art it is and the immediate communication which it has been to generations of readers.

Communications, in other words, may not be dependent on information. Indeed the most perfect communications may be purely "shared experiences" without any logic whatever. Perception has primacy rather than information.

This summary of what we have learned is gross oversimplification. It glosses over some of the most hotly contested issues in psychology and perception. Indeed it may well brush aside most of the issues which the students of learning and of perception, would consider central and important.

But the aim has not been to survey these big areas. My concern here is not with learning or with perception. It is with communications, and in particular, with communications in the large organization, be it business enterprise, government agency, university, or armed service.

This summary might also be criticized for being trite, if not obvious. No one, it might be said, could possibly be surprised at its statements. They say what "everybody knows." But whether this be so or not, it is not what "everybody does." On the contrary, the logical implication for communications in organizations of these apparently simple and obvious statements is at odds with current practice and indeed denies validity to the honest and serious efforts we have been making to communicate for many decades now.

WHY DOWNWARD COMMUNICATIONS CANNOT WORK

What, then, can our knowledge and our experience teach us about communications in organizations, about the reasons for our failures, and about the prerequisites for success in the future?

For centuries we have attempted communication "downward." This, however, cannot work, no matter how hard and how intelligently we try. It cannot work, first, because it focuses on what *we* want to say. It assumes, in other words, that the utterer communicates. But we know that all he does is utter. Communication is the act of the recipient. What we have been trying to do is to work on the emitter, specifically on the manager, the administrator, the commander, to make him capable of being a better communicator. But all one can communicate downward are commands, that is, prearranged signals. One cannot communicate downward anything connected with understanding, let alone with motivation. This requires communication upward, from those who perceive to those who want to reach their perception.

This does not mean that managers should stop working on clarity in what they say or write. Far from it. But it does mean that how we say something comes only after we have learned what to say. And this cannot be found out by "talking to," no matter how well it is being done. "Letters to the Employees," no matter how well done, will be a waste unless the writer knows what employees can perceive, expect to perceive, and want to do. They are a waste unless they are based on the recipient's rather than the emitter's perception.

But "listening" does not work either. The Human Relations School of Elton Mayo, forty years ago, recognized the failure of the traditional approach to communications. Its answer* was to enjoin listening. Instead of starting out with what "we," that is, the executive, want to "get across," the executive should start out by finding out what subordinates want to know, are interested in, are, in other words, receptive to. To this day, the human relations prescription, though rarely practiced, remains the classic formula.

Of course, listening is a prerequisite to communication. But it is not adequate, and it cannot, by itself, work. Listening assumes that the superior will understand what he is being told. It assumes, in other words, that the subordinates can communicate. It is hard to see, however, why the subordinate should be able to do what his superior cannot do. In fact, there is no reason for assuming he can. There is no reason, in other words, to believe that listening results any less in mis-

---

*Especially as developed in Mayo's two famous books, *The Human Problems of an Industrial Civilization* (Harvard Business School, 1933) and *The Social Problems of an Industrial Civilization* (Harvard Business School, 1945).

understanding and miscommunications than does talking. In addition, the theory of listening does not take into account that communications is demands. It does not bring out the subordinate's preferences and desires, his values and aspirations. It may explain the reasons for misunderstanding. But it does not lay down a basis for understanding.

This is not to say that listening is wrong, any more than the futility of downward communications furnishes any argument against attempts to write well, to say things clearly and simply, and to speak the language of those whom one addresses rather than one's own jargon. Indeed, the realization that communications have to be upward—or rather that they have to start with the recipient rather than the emitter, which underlies the concept of listening—is absolutely sound and vital. But listening is only the starting point.

More and better information does not solve the communications problem, does not bridge the communications gap. On the contrary, the more information, the greater is the need for functioning and effective communication. The more information, in other words, the greater is the communications gap likely to be. The information explosion demands functioning communications.

The more impersonal and formal the information process in the first place, the more will it depend on prior agreement on meaning and application, that is, on communications. In the second place, the more effective the information process, the more impersonal and formal will it become; the more will it separate human beings and thereby require separate, but also much greater, efforts, to re-establish the human relationship, the relationship of communication. It may be said that the effectiveness of the information process will depend increasingly on our ability to communicate, and that, in the absence of effective communication—that is, in the present situation—the information revolution cannot really produce information. All it can produce is data.

The information explosion is the most compelling reason to go to work on communications. Indeed, the frightening communications gap all around us—between management and workers; between business and government; between faculty and students, and between both of them and university administration; between producers and consumers, and so on—may well reflect in some measure the tremendous increase in information without a commensurate increase in communications.

WHAT CAN MANAGERS DO?

Can we then say anything constructive about communication? Can we do anything? We can say that communication has to start from the intended recipient of communications rather than from the emitter. In terms of traditional organization we have to start upward. Downward communications cannot work and do not work. They come *after* upward communications have successfully been established. They are reaction rather than action; response rather than initiative.

But we can also say that it is not enough to listen. The upward communications must be focused on something that both recipient and emitter can perceive, focused on something that is common to both of them. They must be focused on what already motivates the intended recipient. They must, from the beginning, be informed by his values, beliefs, and aspirations.

Management by objectives is thus a prerequisite for functioning communication. It requires the subordinate to think through and present to the superior his own conclusions as to what major contribution to the organization—or to the unit within the organization—he should be expected to perform and should be held accountable for.

What the subordinate comes up with is rarely what the superior expects. Indeed, the first aim of the exercise is precisely to bring out the divergence in perception between superior and subordinate. But the perception is focused, and focused on something that is real to both parties. To realize that they see the same reality differently is in itself already communication.

Management by objectives gives to the intended recipient of communication—in this case the subordinate—access to experience that enables him to understand. He is given access to the reality of decision-making, the problems of priorities, the choice between what one likes to do and what the situation demands, and above all, the responsibility for a decision. He may not see the situation the same way the superior does—in fact, he rarely will or even should. But he may gain an understanding of the complexity of the superior's situation and of the fact that the complexity is not of the superior's making, but is inherent in the situation itself.

And these communications, even if they end in a "no" to the subordinate's conclusions, are firmly focused on the aspirations, values, and motivation of the intended recipient. In fact, they start out with the question "What would you *want* to do?" They may then end up with the command "This is what I tell you to do." But at least they force the superior to realize that he is overriding the desires of the subordinate. It forces him to explain, if not to try to persuade. At least he knows that he has a problem—and so does the subordinate.

A performance appraisal based on what a man can do and has done well; or a discussion on a man's development direction, are similarly foundations for communications. They start out with the subordinate's concerns, express his perception, and focus his expectations. They make communications his tool rather than a demand on him.

These are only examples, and rather insignificant ones at that. But perhaps they illustrate the main conclusion to which our experience with communications—largely an experience of failure—and all the work on learning, memory, perception, and motivation point: communication requires shared experience.

There can be no communication if it is conceived as going from the "I" to the "Thou." Communication works only from one member of "us" to another. Communication in organization—and this may be the true lesson of our communication failure and the true measure of our communication need—is not a *means* of organization. It is the *mode* of organization.

Unit II

TECHNICAL SKILLS FOR MANAGEMENT

███

A manager is a person who has specialized knowledge and skills in certain areas. Today's health care manager needs expertise in problem solving, education, and labor relations.

The following three chapters, which deal with the technical skills of management, discuss ways of considering variables that influence decision making while applying educational strategies and promoting positive labor relations in the work environment.

DECISION MAKING

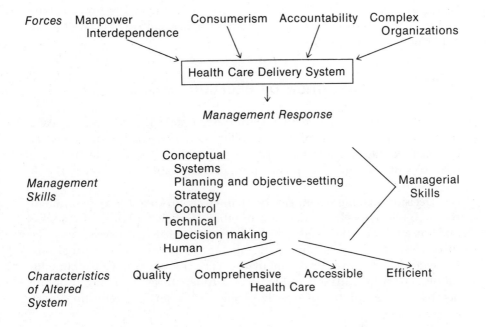

LEARNING OBJECTIVES

After carefully reading this chapter the reader will be able to:
1. Define decision making.
2. List the seven steps in the decision-making process.
3. Define creativity.
4. Define the five steps in the creative process.
5. List the three factors that affect creativity.
6. List the four ways in which a manager creates an effective decision-making process.

INTRODUCTION

Major and minor decision making are daily activities for a manager. Major decisions must be made about the development of patient care programs, which employees will receive raises, and what equipment should be purchased. Minor decisions are made about the best solution for an operating problem, time allocation, and delegation of responsibility and authority.

Regardless of the manner in which problems manifest themselves or the magnitude of the decision, the manager needs specific investigative skills and a thorough understanding of the decision-making process. Furthermore, he needs judgment in selecting the best course of action for the department at a particular time.

DEFINITION OF DECISION MAKING

The management structure within an organization allocates to each supervisor distinct areas of responsibility so that he makes decisions for his part of the organization. He is responsible for coordinating the resources placed under his jurisdiction; decisions about alternative uses of the resources are made constantly.

Decision making, then, can be defined as making a judgment about resource allocation from among a number of choices. This process takes into consideration the needs within the organization, balanced against the forces outside the institution pressing for resources for new programs. For example, the director of ambulatory care chooses to have patient education classes in nutrition rather than a tuberculosis screening program because of the number of elderly people in the service area who do not eat properly.

Decision making clears up organizational problems and facilitates the orderly management of resources by answering basic questions:
1. What are the issues in this situation?
2. What are the major problems associated with these issues?
3. What are the areas that need to be considered?
4. What are the time factors?
5. What are the elements to be measured?
6. How much will it cost?
7. Who will do what?
8. How do the employees feel?

Since decision making is a science and an art, the decision-maker needs both technical and human skills. Insofar as the subject matter can be quantified and programmed, the decision-making activities are scientific. The use of operations research techniques in reducing the waiting time of patients in the outpatient area is an example of application of the scientific aspects of decision making to an operating problem; development of strategies to "sell" the new scheduling procedures to the outpatient department employees illustrates the art of decision making.

Along with sensitivity to the human factors, the use of judgment in decision making is critical. The future is uncertain and can only be approximated. Only through the process of wise discernment, which weighs all of the factors in a situation, can the best decision be obtained. Although the quality of judgment will always vary, better decisions can be made by someone who understands the decision-making process.

POST TEST 6–1

Define decision making.

THE DECISION-MAKING PROCESS

The decision-making process, a complex phenomenon, can best be understood by analyzing each step in the cycle. The eight steps of decision making are illustrated in Figure 12. All of these activities associated with the decision-making process contribute to institutional effectiveness. Three of the activities relate to the problem situation and four to the decision about the problem situation.

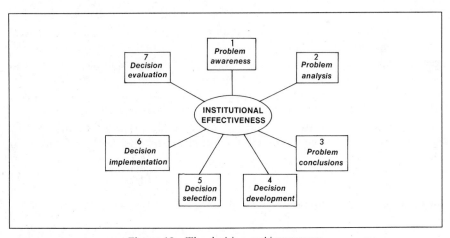

Figure 12   The decision making process

Step 1—Problem Awareness

The three activities involved in problem awareness are environmental monitoring, delineation of the issues surrounding the situation, and the definition of the problem. These are illustrated in Figure 13.

PROBLEM AWARENESS = $\begin{cases} \textit{Environmental Monitoring} \\ \text{Issue Delineation} \\ \text{Problem Definition} \end{cases}$

Figure 13   Problem awareness

ENVIRONMENTAL MONITORING

When the manager is sensitive the the environment and recognizes deviations from the normal course of events, he is able to sense problem situations.

Organizational problems come from a variety of sources—the patients, vendors, community representatives, employees, board members, and union stewards. Effective managers also need a sensitivity to the economic, political, and social forces in the environment that can trigger future problems. Problem awareness, therefore, implies a constant environmental scanning to detect irregularities and a sensitivity to forces that continually affect and change a society.

ISSUE DELINEATION

Awareness of a problem situation implies that the manager can comprehend the real issues and define the problem rather than merely recognize the symptoms of the problem situation. A manager confronted with excessive employee absenteeism might at first glance conclude that he has a scheduling problem; however, after more investigation the real difficulty emerges—the union's attempt at work slowdown prior to a bargaining session. Issues should be stated in the form of questions and should highlight the areas of conflict in thought and feeling relating to the situation.

PROBLEM DEFINITION

The statement of a problem is an essential part of the decision-making process. Unless a problem is put into words, it cannot be analyzed. A comprehensive problem statement includes *what is known, what is unknown,* and *what is sought.*

What is known is usually the manifestation of the problem; what is unknown are the factors causing the problem situation; what is sought are the conditions for the solution of the problem. An example of a problem statement about the absenteeism in the maintenance department is as follows:

> How can employee absenteeism be reduced while insuring ocverage of the department, union contract compliance, and maintenance of employee morale?

This statement can be analyzed further by applying the criteria of what is known, what is unknown, and what is sought:

What is unknown — How can

What is known — employee absenteeism

What is sought — be reduced while insuring coverage of the department, union contract compliance, and maintenance of employee morale?

Step 2 — Problem Analysis

After the problem has been defined, the manager can begin his analysis of it. The four activities associated with this phase of decision making revolve around the definition, collection, and organization of information for decision-making. They are shown in Figure 14.

PROBLEM ANALYSIS =
- *Delineation of areas to be considered*
- *Delineation of elements to be measured*
- *Planning for information retrieval*
- *Collecting and classifying data*

Figure 14   Problem analysis.

DELINEATION OF AREAS TO BE CONSIDERED

The problem definition usually clarifies areas that should be investigated before the solution to a problem can be obtained. For example, in the problem definition cited earlier, "How can employee absenteeism be reduced while insuring coverage of the department, union contract compliance, and maintenance of employee morale?", the areas that should be investigated are absenteeism figures, staffing quotas, the union contract, and factors of employee morale.

DELINEATION OF ELEMENTS TO BE MEASURED

The elements that need to be measured are specified for each area being considered. These elements are facts about the particular area under investigation. The elements that would be documented under absenteeism are as follows:

1. Absenteeism by month for a period of time.
2. Departmental absenteeism against total absenteeism.
3. Absenteeism by employee.
4. Absenteeism of this department against that of a comparable department elsewhere in the city.

PLANNING FOR INFORMATION RETRIEVAL

After the facts that have to be collected are specified, a schedule for the retrieval of this information should be devised. Planning the sequencing of information retrieval guards against information gaps.

COLLECTION AND CLASSIFICATION OF DATA

The facts that have been collected about a segment of the problem should then be organized in such a way that relationships among data can be seen. Graphs, charts, and statistical computations are aids in accomplishing this part of the problem analysis.

Step 3 — Problem Conclusions

When the information has been put into an orderly format and analyzed, the manager can then begin to draw some conclusions from the data. For example, after looking at the absenteeism information, the manager might conclude that the peak months for high absenteeism are July and December. Furthermore, there are only two employees who consistently use all of their allotted sick time.

Step 4 — Decision Development

When the problem has been thoroughly researched, alternative ways of solving the situation can be developed. It is necessary that all possible alternatives be considered. The steps to insure this are shown in Figure 15.

DECISION DEVELOPMENT = *Enlist participation*
Generate ideas
Develop criteria for decision

Figure 15   Decision development.

ENLIST PARTICIPATION

The development of various solutions to problems is one of the most creative parts of the decision-making process. At this stage, the manager should consider participation and multiple inputs from a variety of people within the organization. Soliciting ideas from the people who will have to implement the final decision contributes to an effective strategy.

GENERATE IDEAS

A decision is only as good as the alternatives generated. Several techniques for producing multiple solutions are used by managers. Two of these are brainstorming and the use of advocate teams.

Brainstorming. The basic idea behind brainstorming is that many times critical judgment by others prevents people from expressing unorthodox ideas. In a brainstorming session, a climate that is most conducive to the production of ideas is set up. First, no judgment or evaluation is allowed at all; secondly, the participants are encouraged to produce as many ideas as possible; third, the greater the number of ideas, the better; and finally, combination and improvement of ideas are sought. In addition to contributing ideas of their own, participants should suggest how ideas of others could be used to an advantage or how two or more ideas could be joined into still another idea.

After all the ideas have been produced, they can be evaluated. Critical judgment can be applied after the ideas have been generated.

Use of Advocate Teams. In the advocate-team method, individuals are assigned to groups. Each group then develops a solution. The groups present their idea to a convergence team, usually composed of experts in the area. The members of this team then take all of the solutions, blend and refine them, and present the best solution for the problem.

DEVELOP CRITERIA FOR DECISION SELECTION

In order to make an intelligent decision about the best solution to a problem, criteria need to be developed. Each solution is then evaluated against these standards. The criteria are usually tailormade to fit the particular problem situation and often reflect the values of the manager.

One way of developing criteria is to weigh the advantages and disadvantages of each choice. These pros and cons can then be evaluated in terms of their importance and immediacy.

Another method of evaluating alternatives is to look at them in relation to the goals of the organization. How well does this decision relate to the objectives of the institution? the department? For example, a decision to fire all the employees who have excessive absent days might run contrary to union procedures and interfere with patient care.

A third method of evaluating solutions is look at them against the criteria of suitability, feasibility, and acceptability.

Suitability refers to the accomplishment of objectives.

Will the solution work?
Is it a permanent or interim solution?

Feasibility refers to the implementation of the solution.

Can the organization afford this solution?
What are the risks involved in this solution?
How will the solution affect patient care?

Acceptability refers to the approval of the solution by others.

Will the employees support the decision?
Will the upper management accept the solution?

Step 5 — Decision Selection

The choice among alternatives is difficult. Occasionally, one clearly superior solution will stand out at the conclusion of the testing process. However, usually this is not the case — no one solution has come through all of the evaluations with flying colors.

The best solution will frequently be a combination of two or more solutions. Such a solution is generally adequate and workable under all circumstances.

Step 6 — Decision Implementation

The choice of a solution is not the end of the decision-making process. A plan to implement the decision has to be developed. The steps in this process are shown in Figure 16.

$$\text{DECISION IMPLEMENTATION} = \begin{cases} \textit{Organization of plan for implementation} \\ \textit{Coordination with previous plans} \\ \textit{Communication of the decision} \end{cases}$$

Figure 16   Decision implementation.

ORGANIZATION OF PLAN FOR IMPLEMENTATION

A plan to implement the decision has to be developed. Such questions as the materials, manpower, and money that will be needed to effect this decision need to be explored. How much authority and responsibility should be delegated? Will a new organization be needed to implement the decision? This is one of the most critical aspects of the process, because if the organizational features of the decision implementation are not clearly addressed, the problem situation may remain viable.

COORDINATION WITH PREVIOUS PLANS

The manager should be aware that decisions are interrelated, just as departments of the health facility are dependent on one another. The effective manager considers the impact of the decision on his department, on other departments, and on the organization as a whole and coordinates his decision with previous plans and programs.

In implementing the decision, the manager should guard against duplication of programs or specialized manpower; hence, when possible, solutions to problems should be integrated into existing programs, data systems, and control procedures.

COMMUNICATION OF THE DECISION

A decision is useless if no one is informed about it. The decision and the plan for implementation should be shared by all who are affected by it. Ideally, the employee groups will have been notified of the decision and told how it will be carried out. Other groups, such as department heads, patients, outside groups, and top management, who are peripheral to the decision but affected by it, should also be informed.

Failure to communicate a decision properly can cause resistance to any type of change. If people who will be affected are involved throughout the entire decision-making process, there will be less need to "sell" the solution.

Step 7 — Decision Evaluation

If the problem situation disappears, the solution was a good one. However, there are other ways of monitoring a decision to see whether it is effective.

An elevation system should provide sufficient information to the decision-maker to determine the effectiveness of the decision and the adequacy of its implementation. Some of the key questions an evaluation system answers are as follows:

1. To what extent has the problem situation disappeared?
2. What is the effect of the decision on
   a. the employees?
   b. the patients?
   c. the other departments?
3. Was this an effective decision?
4. What is the total cost of the decision?

POST-TEST 6–2

Mary Engles, the director of the pharmacy at Alma Hospital, has been on the job for two weeks. She was hired because of her previous experience as assistant director of a pharmacy. The other personnel in the pharmacy include one registered pharmacist and four technicians.

Max Schuler, the registered pharmacist, appears uncooperative and lazy. He has told other people in the hospital that he resents working for a woman. Recently, he has been spending a great deal of time at the nursing stations recounting the mistakes Ms. Engles has made since her arrival. Max has been with the hospital for 13 years and manifests a vast knowledge of hospital pharmacy. He was not offered the department head position because he repeatedly told the hospital administrator he did not want to be a manager. He would, however, like to do some additional work in biochemistry at the local university.

Today Ms. Engles received a personal evaluation form for Mr. Schuler. This type of evaluation is done prior to salary increases. The deadline for turning in the form is three days.

Using the practice case, apply the seven steps of the problem-solving and decision-making process to determine a course of action for Ms. Engles.

CREATIVE DECISION-MAKING

Definition of Creativity

A successful manager needs skill in exercising sound judgment before making plans and decisions. This is done by weighing the facts and showing skepticism about unsubstantiated opinions and suggestions. Unfortunately, this necessary skill of critical thinking can stifle the creative expression of new ideas. New ways of looking at existing problems and solutions are also needed by the manager. Creativity is essential if people in work environments are to adapt to the challenges springing from scientific and technological progress. People are beginning to realize that creativity can be cultivated and that the strecthing of the self is one of the most exciting possibilities for a human being. Creativity can be developed if a manager understands the creative process and the conditions that foster this new way of viewing the world.

Creativity is the ability to be aware of the essence of a subject and then to respond to it in a new way. A creative idea goes beyond the established order of things that are clearly determined and accepted and brings new association to existing elements.

Creative people have the ability to be aware of, puzzled by, and responsive to the environmert. They can concentrate and relate to the world around them. Creative minds look for unexpected likenesses and find new combinations of existing realities. They can tolerate conflict and tension and manifest a willingness to begin fresh each day.

POST-TEST 6–3

Define Creativity.

Creative Process

Investigation of the creative cycle reveals that the process is a slow, selective procedure relating to what belongs and what does not belong in a situation. Managers should realize that new ideas are seldom conceived minutely and clearly right at the beginning of the creative process. The development of the idea is gradual, frequently elusive, and, at times, groping. The creative cycle can best be explained by describing the five steps in the process: environmental scanning, probing, development, illumination, and confirmation. The interaction of these elements is illustrated in Figure 17.

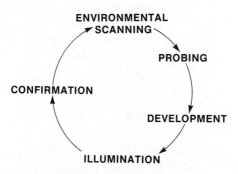

Figure 17   The creative cycle.

ENVIRONMENTAL SCANNING

Sensitivity to the world around us uncovers potential problems and opportunities. Creative skills enable the manager to sense a disturbing element or disequilibrium in the environment. Often a budding problem is masked by occasional tension or discontinuity of the work cycle. Often it is overtly manifested through absenteeism and lowered morale. A creative person who is in tune with the external environment can tell when the elements of the work situation are not in balance.

PROBING

In the second step, the creative manager seeks the facts about the disturbing situation. He assembles in his mind data concerning the problem. Probing assists the mind in collecting the necessary information, which then can be sorted, rearranged, and brought into new associations that will facilitate understanding of the problem in relation to the environment. In collecting information, experts agree that it is better to collect too many facts than too few. This can be done by exhausting all possible sources of information. The creative individual talks to people who at first glance seem to have no bearing on the problem situation but who often can shed light on the matter. After a large amount of information has been collected, it should be organized in such a way that the subtle relationships that point to further insights can be obtained.

DEVELOPMENT

This step, known as the quiet period in the creative cycle, is the time given to mulling all of the facts. It is also a time of apparent inactivity but a period when the subconscious mind directs itself to problems that are of interest to the conscious mind. This time should not be rushed; rather it should be cultivated. Often when people are pondering a problem, they do something entirely different for a while such as gardening, walking, painting, or traveling. During this period, the unconscious does not relax but explores freely through its stored data, sorting and rearranging it until a solution is suggested in a quiet manner.

ILLUMINATION

The solution comes. A new idea is born. Like a flash of light, the way is clear and is transmitted from the unconscious to the conscious. This period of the creative cycle is probably the most exciting, because the product of the effort can be an entirely new approach to an existing problem or an entirely new relationship to elements taken for granted. Often the solution comes when the person least expects it, and it is a good idea to carry a pencil and paper so that when the idea flashes, it can be captured before it disappears.

The acceptance of solutions as they come from the unconscious while the manager is working on the idea is a tricky business. One has to resist the increasing pressure of criticism and judgment of the emerging idea. Critical judgment at this point will inhibit the forward movement of the idea.

CONFIRMATION

This period of activity aims at validating the solution proposed by the unconscious mind. The mind sets about by a logical method or through experimentation to prove or disprove the solution that has been suggested.

In confirmation, it is essential to maintain an open mind so as to avoid rejecting an idea only because of previous approaches to the problem situation. New ideas are worthless until they come into full form and are available for consideration by those who use them.

Sensitivity to the creative cycle enables the manager faced with decision making to let this process develop as problems are investigated and solved. Knowing about creative energy can also give the manager an opportunity to develop this skill in other people.

POST-TEST 6–4

You have been selected to head a special hospital committee that is to study the disposal of the plastic syringes used to give medications. Using the steps of the creative process, develop a new way of disposing of the syringes.

Factors Affecting Creativity

Creativity flourishes in an organization when creativity is rewarded, the tools for creative thinking are available, and managers manifest and expect creativity.

Creative people are sensitive about their innovations. They often are unsure about their idea and need a sympathetic listener. If budding ideas are not squelched before they develop, the creative person is encouraged to pursue the new creation. The best reward for an idea is thoughtful consideration by the manager, followed by honest comments on its potential for implementation. This feedback, coupled with further invitations to think about other problem situations, can do much to stimulate creative action throughout the institution.

Ideas can be generated if the environment provides the resources needed for this process. Examples of possible environmental resources are a library, research laboratories when feasible, creativity training sessions, and a quiet place where a person can sit down and think about a problem in an organized way.

Finally, creativity flourishes when the management team manifests and expects creativity. If a manager understands the creative process, he can do much to encourage creative activities among his staff and the other employees. Since creativity is a matter of many people working together, the imaginative associations produced by these groups are directly related to the ideas and solutions they formulate. Sometimes it is possible to communicate the expectation for creative thinking by letting an employee know in advance that you will visit with him on a specific date and would appreciate some fresh ideas ready for consideration. Another method is to arrange for people engaged in work involving creativity to get away from their offices and families for a two- or three-day retreat. At these "getaways," you can ask, "How can we do this better?"

The creative talents of an organization are its most precious asset. They should be cultivated and conserved so that fresh ways of viewing problems can become the modus operandi.

POST-TEST 6–5

List the three factors that affect creativity.

EFFECTIVE DECISION-MAKING

The manager's participation in decision making is crucial and never-ending. A manager creates effective decision-making processes by telling the institutional story, clarifying communication channels, improving human relations, and developing the decision-making skills described earlier in this chapter.

Telling the Institutional Story

It is naive to assume that all the employees of a department know the objectives and goals of the organization. Frequently, there is misunderstanding about the purpose of the institution, its priorities, and the means by which objectives will be attained.

Specifying the institutional goals and objectives is not an easy task. However, only if it is done and is accompanied by clear policies and time tables for the accomplishment of the goals can the thrust of the organization be known and decision making facilitated.

Decisions are made in light of the goals of the organization. Usually, in the objectives-definition stage, the problems of the institution are examined and objectives formulated in response to them. Once the friction points are known and analyzed, problem situations can be anticipated and solved more efficiently. Familiarity with the goals and objectives of the institution promotes unity of effort among employees, which heightens employee morale.

Clarification of Communication Channels

Information is the medium for decision making. It must be obtained and classified and conveyed to everyone who needs it.

Unless a manager knows what is going on in the organization, problems can get out of hand. The leader in the small, face-to-face organization has a great advantage over the bureaucratic leader because he has on-the-spot sensitivity for what is taking place. The manager is a large institution is more likely to rely on reports, existing policies, and miscellaneous observations.

The effective decision-maker has to be aware of not only what is taking place but also of what should be occurring but is not. He should continually be sensitive to what people know and feel about the organization and their part in it.

Many think of organizational communication as a process involving letters, memoranda, regulations, and similar documents. It is all this, and more. It includes conversations, gestures, expressions, and attitudes. Applied organizationally, it involves all that affects the exchange of information and ideas between people, and it usually occurs through established organizational channels within the institution.

Communication problems that affect decision making occur when the specified channels of communication are not followed. Such is the case when the news of an increase in patients' falling from beds on Ward 3E never reaches the nursing office, or when housekeeping employees' complaints about their working conditions are unknown to the personnel director.

Information that could be used for decision making should also be available to managers. Procedure and policy manuals, personnel handbooks, and back copies of memos and bulletin are of great use.

Improving Human Relations

Decision making is enhanced when it is supported by people who have been involved in the problem-solving and decision-making processes.

As the work culture continues to stress the dignity and importance of the individual, the worker will demand more knowledge of and participation in matters affecting him. Unity of purpose flourishes in the presence of a free flow of information. Confusion is reduced if the employees are told what is being done and why.

There is growing acceptance of the fact that everyone in the organization contributes to its effectiveness. People in the operating situations should be consulted about problem situations. Often the night porter has a better idea about the best type of cleaning equipment than does an assistant administrator, and frequently he is just as concerned about the cost as is the controller. His judgment is of value in dealing with the subjects he knows so intimately; it is management's loss when this point is not understood.

There are many ways by which personnel at all levels can be involved. The simplest, most direct, and probably the best of these is to ask the employees' advice. This can come about most easily in normal day-to-day relationships. It should be emphasized that if advice is asked, it will have to be followed, at least a part of the time, or the employees will feel that they are being compromised.

A proper knowledge of what is going on in the organization will invariably underscore the importance of the individual in it. Even the simplest of operations will be seen to involve others, both directly and indirectly.

The manager should understand not only what the individual does but also how he views his role. What are his personal standards of accomplishment? What does he hope to become? How does he see his current assignment relating to his long-run objectives? Who makes up his peer group? How do they evaluate him? Sensitivity to these human concerns can simplify problem-solving and produce the best possible decision.

POST-TEST 6–6

List the ways a manager creates an effective decision-making process.

SUMMARY

Decision making is a judgment about resource allocation from among a number of alternatives. It comprises problem awareness, analysis, and conclusions; and decision development, selection, implementation, and evaluation. Decision making is enhanced through creativity, clear communication channels, and effective human relations.

RECAP EXERCISE 6

As director of admissions, Mrs. Carter is responsible for the work of approximately 35 employees, 20 of whom were classified as intake workers or file clerks. Acting under pressure from Mr. Brown, the administrator, she agreed to allow the McGee Consulting Firm to enter the admissions office to make a time-study and work-method analysis in an effort to improve the efficiency and output of the staff.

The consultants began their study by observing and recording each detail of the work of the intake workers and clerks. After two days of observation, they indicated that they were prepared to begin their time study on the following day.

The next morning, five of the office employees participating in the study were absent. On the following day, ten employees were absent. In concern, Mrs. Carter investigated the cause of the absenteeism by telephoning several absentees. Each employee related approximately the same story. Each was nervous, tense, and physically tired, after being viewed as a "guinea pig" for several days. One woman told Mrs. Carter that her physician had advised her to ask for a leave of absence if working conditions were not improved.

Shortly after the telephone calls, the chief of the systems analysis team explained to Mrs. Carter that if there were as many absences on the next day, his team would have to drop the study and proceed to another department. He elaborated that a scientific analysis would be impossible to formulate with ten employees absent. Realizing that she would be held responsible for the failure of the systems analysis, Mrs. Carter began to create alternative courses of action that would provide the conditions necessary for the study.

Using the steps of the decision-making process,

1. What is the most creative solution to this situation? Use the steps in the decision-making process to come up with your answer.

2. What steps should be taken in the organization to ensure that this does not happen in other departments?

REFERENCES

1. Barnard, C. I.: *The Functions of the Executive.* Cambridge, Mass., Harvard University Press, 1938.
2. Brenkers, Henry S. (ed.): *Decision Making: Creativity, Judgment and Systems.* Columbus, Ohio State University Press, 1972.
3. DiVincenti, Marie: *Administering Nursing Service.* Boston, Little, Brown & Co., 1972.
4. Hamilton, James A.: *Decision Making in Hospital Administration and Medical Care.* Minneapolis, University of Minnesota Press, 1967.
5. Holloman, C. R., and Hendrick, H. W.: Problem solving in different sized groups. *Personnel Psychology, 24*:489–500, 1971.
6. Kepner, C. H., and Tregoe, B. B.: *The Rational Manager: A Systematic Approach to Problem Solving and Decision Making.* New York, McGraw-Hill Book Co., 1965.
7. Kobayashi, Shigern: *Creative Management.* New York, American Management Association, 1971.
8. Miller, James R.: *Professional Decision Making.* New York, Praeger Publishers, 1970.
9. Morton, Michael S.: *Management Decision Systems — Computer Based Support for Decision Making.* Boston, Harvard Business School, 1971.
10. Perrow, C.: Hospitals: technology, structure, and goals. In March, J. G. (ed.): *Handbook of Organizations.* Chicago, Rand-McNally, 1965, pp. 910–971.
11. Rausch, Erwin: *Decision Making.* Chicago, Science Research Association, Inc., 1968.
12. Taylor, Calvin W.: *Climate for Creativity.* Elmsford, N. Y., Pergamon Press, 1972.

EDUCATION AND TRAINING

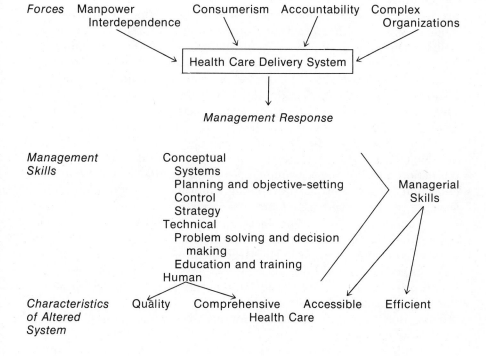

LEARNING OBJECTIVES

After reading this chapter, the reader will be able to:
1. List the three types of educational programs.
2. Define the five steps in the development of education programs.
3. Specify four characteristics of adult learners.

INTRODUCTION

● The cardiologists request a demonstration of the new monitoring equipment.
● The head nurses want to know about collective bargaining techniques.

● The women's auxiliary is planning a session on PSROs.
● The personnel staff thinks the orientation program should be broadened.

Demands for education within the hospital abound. More frequently, department heads are looking for assistance in the organization, financing, and evaluation of educational programs.

Several forces converging on the health field simultaneously have caused this increased emphasis on learning. The knowledge explosion precipitated a proliferation of information about improved treatment modalities and health delivery mechanisms that still continues. It is impossible to keep up with the advances in a subject area without attending lectures, short-term courses, or institutes. The increased emphasis on quality of care through competent manpower has caused the licensing and professional groups to stress continuing education as a condition of relicensure for their members. The recent court dceisions placing the responsibility for the practice of medicine on the hospital have forced administrators to look closely at the skill and competence of their personnel. Finally, the social culture is facilitating a movement toward self-actualization and lifelong learning. In response to this trend, the general educational institutions are developing innovations in education so that learning can be individualized and self-paced.

Although one of the main objectives of hospitals has always been education, the emphasis in this area centered historically on medical and nursing education programs. The large medical centers were the laboratories of clinical experience for student physicians, nurses, and allied health professionals, while selected community hospitals provided internships and residencies to young physicians. Within most hospitals, the nursing department sponsored programs of orientation, skill training, continuing education, and management development for their staff. However, within the past few years, the educational function of the hospitals has broadened to include all hospital personnel, boards of trustees, patients, and community groups.

Much of this educational activity is coordinated at the institutional level through the use of a department of education with a full-time director. However, much education needs to take place in the individual departments under the direction of the department head. It is his responsibility to see that his employees know the goals of the organization and the requirements of their jobs. This training function is imparted through a variety of teaching activities, ranging from on-the-job training to formal group programs.

Several operating problems, such as high turnover rates, accidents, patient complaints, equipment breakdown, and lowered employee productivity, can be corrected through employee educational programs. The purpose of employee education, then, is to help the employee to gain effectiveness in his present or future work through the development of appropriate habits of thought and action. The development of knowledge, skills, and attitudes needed to perform adequately on the job will assist him in actualizing his potential as a person.

TYPES OF EDUCATIONAL PROGRAMS

Hospital educational programs serve three groups—health manpower, consumers, and boards of trustees.

Health Manpower

The health manpower programs comprise preparatory education, inservice education, continuing education, and graduate medical education.

Preparatory education refers to the programs that prepare persons for initial employment in hospitals and other health care agencies. Examples of these are the medical, nursing, dental, allied health professional, and technical programs. The majority of this effort is carried out at the university or college, while the hospital provides the laboratory experience in patient care. These programs are directly supervised by the university faculty. They are usually financed through federal and state subsidies and tuition payments.

In-service education refers to orientation, skill training, and management development.

ORIENTATION. These are programs that acquaint employees with the goals of the institution and the department, personnel benefits and policies, and the particular task or type of work the person will be performing. This type of program is threefold: the orientation to the total institution, to the department, and to the worker unit. The statement of the overall goals and resources of the institution can be given by someone from the personnel or education department. However, the orientations to the department and the work unit are coordinated by the departmental manager. In this phase the new employee "settles in" while becoming acquainted with the purpose of the department, the particular policies and benefits that affect him, and the special knowledge and skills necessary to do his job. This phase of employee education is very important because it gives the new worker a sense of identity and a familiarity with the new institution.

SKILL TRAINING. These programs prepare the employees to function efficiently in their jobs by providing them with an opportunity to learn the necessary skills for operating equipment, performing services, or mastering complicated techniques. Examples of skill training include learning to operate a heart-lung machine, master techniques of operating room protocol, and run a floor-washing machine.

MANAGEMENT DEVELOPMENT. These programs are especially designed to provide the knowledge, attitudes, and skills necessary for those who are in supervisory positions. The subject matter concerns itself with activities of planning, organizing, coordinating, and controlling the resources necessary to deliver patient care in a health facility.

Continuing education programs help health professionals to maintain and improve their particular knowledge and skills. These programs can be conducted within the hospital, developed cooperatively with universities and professional organizations, or carried on outside the hospital. The financing of these programs is determined by the organizational arrangement. Often the hospitals reimburse employees by continuing their salaries while they are attending the program or through tuition rebate mechanisms.

Graduate medical education refers to the specialized residency programs offered in hospitals for physicians who have graduated from medical school and who wish to pursue an area of clinical practice in depth. This is usually done as a cooperative venture between the university and the teaching hospital. These programs are supervised by a director of medical education and can be sponsored by academic medical centers, hospitals affiliated with a medical school, or nonaffiliated free-standing health care institutions. They are financed by grants, endowments, and patient care revenues.

Consumer Education

Consumer education programs meet the needs of patients who want to know more about their conditions and treatments and citizens who want to learn about health practices and the issues affecting health care delivery. Patient education programs are conducted at the patient units and in the clinics and deal with topics related to health maintenance or adjustment of existing conditions. Patient education is viewed more and more as an integral part of all patient treatment and is financed by operating revenues. Other programs offered for consumer groups deal with the questions relating to the organization, governance, and financing of health care. These consumer education programs are conducted by a variety of health professionals within the institution.

Board of Trustee Education

These educational programs are oriented toward providing information about policy matters that have an impact on the overall management of the hospital, such as the legal, organizational, financial, and manpower considerations of decision making in today's health environment. Frequently this information is imparted at board meetings by the administrator, or more formal programs are offered through professional associations.

The role of the manager in these activities varies from that of instructor to facilitator to evaluator of the completed program. When the manager sees education as a management tool, he can use it effectively in the achievement of organizational goals by reducing the time required to bring the inexperienced employee to an acceptable level of job proficiency.

POST-TEST 7–1

1. Define the three types of educational programs conducted within the hospital.
2. Specify the types of educational programs that are necessary for the operation of a hospital program.

DEVELOPMENT OF EDUCATIONAL PROGRAMS

In order to conduct effective educational programs, the manager needs an understanding of the basic steps in the development and implementation of an educational program, whether it be orientation, skill training, continuing education, or management development.

The five components of an educational program are environmental assessment, formulation of objectives, program planning, program implementation, and program evaluation. The interaction of these components is seen in Figure 18.

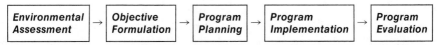

Figure 18 The design and evaluation of educational programs.

Environmental Assessment

Employee education is not an end but a means to an end; it exists only to help achieve organizational goals and objectives. To be effective, this management tool must be used when and where it is needed and not as "window dressing" to impress outsiders about the staff development of the programs offered by the institution.

The use of training to achieve organizational goals requires careful assessment of the learning needs of employees within the hospital. This assessment process then provides a rationale for the determination of objectives. Specifically, it defines the relevant environment, describes the desired and actual conditions pertaining to that environment, identifies unmet needs and unused opportunities, and diagnoses the problems that prevent needs from being met and opportunities from being used.

A major component of the assessment process is the determination of the employee learning needs. This determination involves an understanding of needs as perceived by both the employee and the employer. A training activity or educational program that does not make sense to the employees will not succeed, for they cannot be expected to respond enthusiastically to a new venture unless they believe that it will affect their well-being.

Some of the main questions that are asked during the environmental assessment are the following:

1. What are the institutional needs?
2. What is the institutional setting?
3. What are the goals of the institution?
4. What are the boundaries of the institution?
5. What patient-care and educational programs are already operative?
6. What resources are available for conducting educational programs?
7. What are the major problems in the environment?
8. What are the client needs? The answer to this question involves a study of the various clients of the hospital to see what type of educational programs are needed. These clients are the professional and nonprofessional employees, consumers, patients, and members of the board of trustees.
9. What is the decision-making structure of the institution? This is an important piece of information, since the methods of "getting action" and mobilizing resources have to be known so that the programs can be implemented. In planning new programs, it is a good idea to know who on the administrative staff needs to be kept informed.
10. What are the trends in education, patient care, and management? This question is germane because it focuses on the future and emerging developments that are being planned in these areas. Closed-circuit television can have a decided impact on the development of specialized programs, and primary care will require new skills of the people involved in it. All of these trends should be monitored.

The answers to these questions become the basis of information for the delineation of educational objectives.

Formulation of Objectives

In order for objectives to be meaningful, they should be written in performance terms. A performance objective is a statement that a) clearly gives the conditions under which the student will be evaluated (the situation), b) designates the behavior that the student should display (behavioral term), and c) indicates the minimum level at which the student must perform in order to complete the instructional requirements.

Educational programs need stated objectives to provide a guide for planning the content of the sessions, the teaching strategies, and the evaluation criteria that will be used to assess the performance of the student. A well-written objective, then, contains a situation, the behavioral term, and the acceptance level. An example follows:

the situation—Given a list of four procedures for turning a comatose
        patient

the behavioral term—the student will state

the acceptance level—the two correct procedures. Minimum acceptance
        level is stating one of the correct procedures.

Program Planning

After the objectives have been clearly stated, the educator begins. A planning guide that includes all of the following elements can be used effectively during this phase:

1. the information that an educational program will contain.
2. how the material will be presented.
3. the learning exercises that will be used.
4. the teaching aids that will be used.
5. the consultants who will be used in program development.

Program Implementation

If the program has been well planned, the implementation phase is usually easy. During this period, the instructor monitors the progress of the educational program, how well objectives are being met, and the physical and psychological environment for learning.

Some of the obstacles that could impede the progress of the program are lack of clear communication about the purpose of the educational sessions, lack of equipment and supplies for teaching, course content that is not meeting the needs of the learner, and improper scheduling of the courses.

Some factors that should be considered in the physical environment are pleasant surroundings and well-planned facilities. Classrooms should be removed from work areas because of the noise interference and heavy traffic. Classrooms should be well-lighted and adequately ventilated, with tables and chairs arranged to facilitate interaction. The use of introductions and name badges are helpful to stimulate communication. Finally, the necessary equipment and teaching aids should be available, and the instructor should know how to use them.

Attention should also be given to the psychological environment. Participants should not be afraid to speak but should interact freely. In addition, they should not be punished for making mistakes, and a feeling of comfort and acceptance among the participants should be generated. The instructor should act to make the situation one in which people may speak out, fumble for answers, and argue freely, without embarrassment.

Program Evaluation

Program evaluation refers to the instructor's, the participants', and the supervisor's assessment of the value of an educational activity. Evaluation is done to determine whether the objectives were met and whether the program should be repeated, altered, or terminated. Evaluation is complex and difficult to perform but necessary if the manager or instructor is to determine the progress and final outcome of the program. Evaluation should be seen in the context of continually gathering information about the progress and effectiveness of the educational program.

POST-TEST 7–2

Define the five steps in the development of educational programs.

CHARACTERISTICS OF ADULT LEARNERS

In order to effectively plan educational programs that will be relevant for the employees, professional students, and consumers, it is necessary to understand that adults have different mechanisms for learning than do younger people. When planning learning experiences for adult learners, the following factors should be kept in mind:

1. Adults are self-directed, responsible, and mature. They should take an active role in the planning and development of their programs. They usually are aware of their learning deficiencies and need assistance in finding learning resources. When they actively participate in the development of the learning experience, motivation and interest are high. Likewise, when adults are given a passive role in learning, their interest wanes quickly. For this reason, they should be involved in the development of the objectives and the design of the educational programs. The adult learner should take an active part in diagnosing his learning needs.

He should evaluate his progress toward attaining the stated objectives and be active in the overall conduct of the program.

2. Adults bring life experiences to the learning situation that can be used as a resource for other students and provide a foundation for acquiring new knowledge and skills. In planning learning strategies for employees, the manager should use discussion groups, role playing, and interactive techniques so that the experience of all the members of the group can be shared. The adult learner should be made to feel that he is a resource for the other people in the group.

3. Adults relate to complex problems in their work and social situation. Therefore, learning is enhanced when new knowledge is used to solve the problems in their immediate reality. Problem-solving exercises and pragmatic discussions excite and keep the interest of the adult learner.

4. Adults need immediate feedback on their work so that further learning can be facilitated. Reinforcement during discussions and class assignments reassures the person that he is understanding the information correctly or indicates that he should work harder to develop the knowledge and skills being discussed.

POST TEST 7–3

Specify four characteristics of adult learners.

SUMMARY

The manager increasingly uses education and training as a means of upgrading the effectiveness of his employee group. One should understand the relationship of a departmental educational function to the health institution as a whole. Likewise the process of developing, implementing, and evaluating educational programs is essential if the manager wishes to motivate his employees to continually learn.

RECAP EXERCISE 7

Myra Block has been in charge of the physical therapy department for the past two months. During that time she has made a list of the problem areas that she would like to correct in her department. Some of the problems she has identified are the following:

1. Physical therapy employees do not know anything about the other departments of the hospital.

2. Three members of the professional staff would like to upgrade their knowledge and skills in the use of the hydrotherapy machines.

3. The three supervisors in the department would like to know more about budgeting and construction.

4. Many of the patients who are using crutches have asked for classes in crutch walking. Ms. Block also thinks that there are other patient education programs that would be beneficial, such as gait training and back exercises.

The personnel department has recently started an educational division and will be initiating a hospital-wide orientation program soon.

1. Decide how each of these educational needs should be met.

2. List the steps that should be considered in planning the patient education programs.

REFERENCES

1. Argyris, Chris: *Management and Organizational Development.* New York, McGraw-Hill Book Co., 1972.
2. Bergevin, P.: *A Philosophy for Adult Education.* New York, Seabury Press, 1967.
3. Hospital Research and Educational Trust: Planning programs for the adult learner. *Bull. Hosp. Educ. Training,* July, 1968.
4. Hospital Research and Educational Trust: The process of evaluation and follow-up in training. *Bull. Hosp. Educ. Training,* November, 1968.
5. Hospital Research and Educational Trust: *Correspondence Education and the Hospital.* Chicago, HRET, 1969.
6. Lerdo, L., and Cross, L.: Performance-oriented training-results, management and follow-up. *J. Am. Soc. Training Directors, 16*:19, 1962.
7. Magner, Monica M.: *Inservice Education Manual.* St. Louis, Catholic Hospital Association, 1974.
8. McTerna, Edmund J., and Hawkins, Robert O., Jr. (eds.): *Educating Personnel for the Allied Health Professions and Services: Administrative Considerations.* St. Louis, C. V. Mosby Co., 1972.
9. Nader, Leonard: *Developing Human Resources.* Houston, Gulf Publishing Co., 1970.
10. Otto, Calvin P., and Glaser, Rollin O.: *The Management of Training.* Reading, Mass., Addison-Wesley Publishing Co., 1970.
11. Saint, Avice: *Learning at Work.* Chicago, Nelson-Hall Company, 1974.
12. Tracey, William R.: *Designing Training and Development Systems.* New York, American Management Association, 1971.
13. Tracey, William R.: *Managing Training and Development Systems.* New York, American Management Association, 1971.
14. Weigand, James E. (ed.): *Developing Teacher Competencies.* Englewood Cliffs, N.J., Prentice-Hall, Inc., 1971.

LABOR RELATIONS

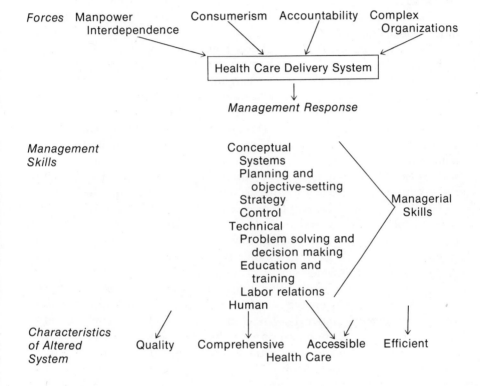

LEARNING OBJECTIVES

After reading this chapter, you will be able to:

1. Define the concept of exchange.

2. Apply the exchange concept to management-employee relationships.

3. Define four types of exchange relationships.

4. State three environmental and societal factors that are causing an increase in unionization of employees.

5. State five elements of a positive employee-management relations program.

INTRODUCTION

The relative importance of employee-management relations increases as more hospitals and other health-care organizations encounter difficulties in obtaining competent employees and, more recently, as unions request recognition as bargaining agents for employees. Various changes in our society and in the health care industry contribute to this historical reassessment of how employees in hospitals will relate to the management of health-care services.

Basically, employees have always engaged in an exchange relationship with employing organizations; unions and other types of employee groups represent devices to strengthen and professionalize the bargaining relationship. While union organizations may be relatively new to the health-care field, they too are organizations, albeit specialized, with goals and objectives, methods for achieving them, and all of the problems of insuring that their owner-members receive appropriate benefits from contributions made. Insight into the needs, desires, and wants of employees will provide the manager with the opportunity to more effectively balance the organization's needs for work accomplishments with employee desire to benefit from and contribute to the work effort. Irrespective of how these employee needs find expression, an understanding of them gives the manager insight into how to maintain a positive employee-relation stance that will both gain acceptance from employees and contribute to organizational effectiveness.

Because many variables that affect the behavior of people remain beyond the manager's control, conflicts will occur with or without unionization. For example, strivings for equal rights for blacks contributed to the mobilization and unionization of black hospital workers. Few managers could have or would have wanted to stem this motivation to achieve equality. However, other things being equal, health-care organizations with good employee relations programs seem less likely to be unionized or to face heavy conflict when unionized.

The suggestions or recommendations for manager action made throughout this section of the book should always be carefully considered to insure its appropriateness to a particular situation. Behavioral science research indicates that appropriate action is contingent upon a variety of circumstances. For example, involving employees in goal-setting and decision-making makes sense in housekeeping and other more routine tasks. It may be less appropriate during a neurosurgical procedure. Consultation helps when employee expertise exceeds manager expertise. However, in a rapidly unfolding emergency, managers may be forced to decide something immediately even if the best solution could have been reached by more deliberative means.

EXCHANGE AND EMPLOYEE RELATIONS

The notion of exchange, or of giving one thing for another, permeates social and organizational life. In earlier times, goods and services often moved in direct exchange between people. Doctors in some areas still receive goods or services in lieu of dollars for their services. For the most part, however, our complex economy operates without the direct transfer of goods and services among the parties who make up our specialized society.

Money exchanges between health care organizations and employees play a major role in the rendering of services by an employee and the utilization of services by the organization. Other less tangible but important social rewards also flow from the work relationship. Affiliation with a prestigious organization or a well-liked group or profession can enhance the benefit of association for an employee, just as association with work of lower status, internally or externally, can reduce the benefit felt from the relationship.

Life in the work place provides many illustrations of exchange relationships. A simple "Well done" usually brings forth a "Thank you." If the task performed went beyond what might be routinely expected and went unnoticed—or worse, was seen but unacknowledged by the supervisor—the worker might not complain or remark the omission but may nevertheless hesitate to perform beyond the normal in the future. Common courtesies constitute important exchange mechanisms. Consistent contributions beyond expectations or "norms" deserve further consideration. For example, persons consistently taking on the toughest task, volunteering for unusual assignments, or getting more done during the work period than others will and should expect some acknowledgment beyond the usual thank you. Merit increases, promotions, and transfers to higher paying and or more prestigious jobs often must be considered. In spite of this obvious fact, many times busy people will overlook what is happening around them and miss otherwise obvious contributions leading to hurt feelings and occasional retributions by the employee.

In order to test your own situation, list the employees who report directly to you and answer the following questions:

1. Does this person always perform in the expected fashion? or perhaps above the average or even below? Have you recently acknowledged these facts, verbally, in writing, or otherwise?

2. Do I routinely ask this person how things are going to detect both problems and outstanding performance? Is there a mutually understood level of performance expectation?

3. When might I get together with this employee to discuss work activities? What should be brought up at that meeting?

Periodic assessments of this type will assist the supervisor in becoming more alert to opportunities for balancing the organization's response to employee contributions.

Although exchange relationships appear relatively simple, they may be more complex than an inquiring manager or researcher can easily discern. The simple notion of "you scratch my back and I'll scratch yours" misses some important considerations. Persons with great prestige or other economic or political resources may always be able to assist others without allowing or permitting others to return the favor. While the initial favors may evoke gratitude, continued inability to reciprocate can lead to feelings of inferiority and hostility toward the giver. What may seem fair in one organization may be compared with other settings known to the participants. Think for a moment about relations you have had with others. Is there someone who continually befriends you but never allows you to reciprocate? Or is there someone to whom you often offer or provide aid but who has not been able or allowed to do some favor for you in return? Such relationships often get out of balance and lead to feelings of hostility.

Also, the mere addition of one type of unit of exchange (money, for example) may produce less satisfaction than some other less tangible good or even a reduced workload. Moreover, for each type of unit of exchange—money, working conditions, opportunity to meet personal goals, control over one's own destiny, and a host of other factors—there are multiple considerations that must be taken into account in determining the equity of the exchange. Consider some of the "exchanges" that you have made recently. Were they equitable? Did the other party perceive them to be so? What evidence do you have for this feeling? You might use the same employee list and go over these questions in relation to each just to check your "balance sheet."

Inevitably, our expectations about what others will view as being valuable hinge upon assumptions that we make, either implicitly or explicitly. For example, the administrator could assume that if the pathologist is given more automated equipment in the laboratory, greater volume and more diverse testing can be obtained.

The assumptions here include availability of automated equipment, sufficient number of cases to justify purchase of the equipment, sufficient physician interest in a variety of tests, and a possible interest of the pathologist in research. Alternatively, the volume of work for the pathologist may be insufficient to fully utilize the resources available, in which case the administrator might encourage arrangements with other institutions to buy part of the pathologist's time, allowing for a possible reduction in expense to the hospital while increasing the pathologist's income and satisfaction. The exchange would allow for a net increase in value to both parties, as well as provide for overall improved utilization of resources for the community.

Questioning one's original assumptions often provides insight into the nature of the opportunity or problem originally presented.

POST-TEST 8–1

1. Define the concept of exchange.
2. Hospitals are one of the more complex types of health care delivery organizations and employ or utilize the skills of a variety of workers. If you were asked to consider designing a reward structure that would encourage each of the types of personnel listed below to contribute more to the hospital, what types of exchanges would you consider?

	Salary Increase	Shift Change	Promotion	Job Transfer	Technical Assistance
Neurosurgeon					
Pathologist					
Assistant administrator					
Coronary-care unit nurse					
Dietary employee— tray person (60 years old)					
Admitting clerk (22 years old)					
Security guard (44 years old, male, father of four)					

TYPES OF EXCHANGE UNITS

The exchange process occurs through various organizational mechanisms such as wages, seniority, appreciation and respect, and equity.

Wages

Wages and other economic incentives may not be the only unit of exchange in employee-management relationships, but their importance with low- and middle-income workers should not be dismissed lightly. The value of the economic exchange offered by the organization in return for the workers' contributions will be influenced by a variety of factors.

COMMUNITY WAGE LEVEL

The general wage level in the community provides one of the guideposts by which workers gauge the relative value of their wages. For some workers, receiving wages similar to those received by persons doing similar work in the same community constitutes an important consideration. For others, whose skills or other factors such as age or marital status make them more mobile, the wages paid for similar work in other areas or communities may be relatively more important. In general, the more specialized and more highly educated personnel will view their salaries in relation to a broader labor market both within the local area and in the larger arena in which they compete for work. While non-wage considerations (e.g., marriage, family) may keep skilled people in local labor markets at noncompetitive rates, the employing organizations risk higher levels of dissatisfaction with this type of inequity.

The reference community might be thought of in several ways. In a large city, neighborhoods, inner-city, suburbs, and other such divisions might constitute reference communities for wage purposes; in rural areas and small towns, the entire area would offer a reference base for comparison.

The internist in private practice and the internist engaged in teaching and research within a medical school, assuming that both have become well established in their own setting, seem likely to have different reference communities. While both will undoubtedly be somewhat aware of incomes for similar pursuits nationally, the private practitioner will be more closely tied to the local income comparison. To the extent that his income depends upon the network of clientele and referrals personally established, part of his skills-for-hire depends upon the local base and are not transferable. The teacher/researcher based at a medical school depends less on local clientele than on his teaching and research skills, which can more easily be transferred to other locations, thus making his reference community other medical schools in the United States. For nurses, a similar comparison can be made. At the other extreme, the housekeeper can usually find other local employment in schools, offices, and hotels.

WAGE LEVELS WITHIN THE ORGANIZATION AND AMONG OCCUPATIONS

People also compare and contrast their wages for work with other occupations within their own profession and other levels within organizations. Registered nurses on night duty will probably consider wages for day duty, intensive care, operating-room nursing positions, and home care and public health. At the same time, nursing salaries compared with other occupational groups within the same organization also constitute reference points. Additional contributing factors include difficulty of work, sex, and mobility opportunities for people in the particular occupation.

Seniority

Relative wage levels become differentiated because of various factors. Time in the position or with the organization often result in somewhat higher wages for persons whose contributions differ little from those of younger workers with less service. Experience and depth of understanding, which normally come with seasoning on the job, may contribute to better production. To the extent that great disparities exist in the performance of senior workers, and even more among junior staff where seniority pay differentials exist, friction and dissatisfaction may result.

At the other end of the time-on-the-job and age spectrum, younger workers may prefer to sacrifice short-run wages if opportunities exist to learn and develop more desirable or valuable skills that would soon lead to higher wages and status. However, they may be less likely to postpone wages, for, say, higher pension benefits, which would be realized only after decades of waiting. In general, this type of trading off between today's contribution and tomorrow's opportunity must be monitored both in overall plans and in individual counseling and work assignment situations. For example, would you plan a different benefit wage package for a work group in which 80 per cent are married, middle-aged women than for a work group in which 80 per cent are unmarried women and a few older workers? In general, the younger women would be expected to seek higher short-run benefits, with less concern for acquiring seniority and pension rights. Some of the group would wish for excellent training and experimental opportunities to build into better careers, while others would be using the job for income while looking toward marriage and the raising of families in the longer run. If you build your plan around one type, it may not attract the other. However, if the labor market permits, you may wish to make the job attractive to one type or the other.

Appreciation and Respect

In their interactions with others, people need many things that go beyond the usual and explicit employee-organization relationship. Appreciation as an individual and a contributing member of the organization seems basic yet often is not mentioned in employment contracts. Establishment of a pleasant working climate and a positive relationship with workers can and does occur under a wide variety of conditions. Even the proverbial slave driver can be fair and consistent in correcting workers on performance and procedure. At the same time, the "good" boss may overlook the variations in performance of some for fear of hurting them, ignoring the fact that such neglect leads to less than optimal performance and thereby injures the individuals involved and the reputation of the boss. In seeking ways to improve performance, remember that the employee with exceptional knowledge, skill, technique, and attitude can be demoralizing both to himself and to his colleagues and that individual or collective attitudes may need correction.

Equity

Equity in rotation of assignments, praise when due, and status symbols can and often do add to an attractive or even an unattractive economic benefit-wage package. Uniform colors, types, and styles can take on great significance, especially in the medical world. For example, consider the following situations and sketch out a positive approach in dealing with each.

1. A housekeeping employee leaves streaks when mopping floors.
2. A ward clerk says no and hangs up the telephone when a caller asks whether the head nurse is available.
3. A secretary is often late and frequently absent from work.

In approaching these dilemmas, first analyze the problem. The employee may fail to recognize the necessity of keeping the department functioning smoothly and seeking help from the supervisor when work does not go well. Second, the employee may lack a systematic plan for doing and completing work in a superior fashion. Third, competing interests, either outside the job or within the organization, may lead to the relative neglect of some aspects of one's direct personal responsibilities.

Each of the above-cited instances could be the result of lack of incentive or motivation, or lack of knowledge of appropriate procedures. More likely the problems stem from a variety of interrelated causes.

Several remedies could be considered. First, specific policies related to the expected performance should be developed fairly and promptly observed and implemented. Second, you should attempt to find out all of the possible causes—personal and otherwise—of each incident. You might start by asking "Could you explain. . . ?" Corrective suggestions and possibly a statement of the consequences for not complying should follow, provided you can enforce such a statement.

Explain the problems that arise from failure to carry out policy and correct procedure. The importance of reliable and effective performance should be pointed out without threatening specific penalties. However, if there is repeated failure, the supervisor should be certain that expecta-

---

POST-TEST 8–2

1. Define four types of exchange relationships.
2. What areas would the following workers be likely consider in determining whether their wages were similar to others in their field?

	National	Regional	Local
Registered nurse			
Housekeeping employee			
Carpenter			
Internist — medical-school-based			
Internist — private practitioner			
Administrator			
Director of nurses			
Secretary			

---

tions and consequences for failure are both understood and recorded, in case further repeats lead to disciplinary action.

ENVIRONMENTAL AND SOCIETAL FACTORS CONTRIBUTING TO UNIONIZATION OF EMPLOYEES

Continuing changes in our society influence how workers, both professional and supportive, view their relations with employers. Changes in the status and aspirations of different groups, the changing role of government in the delivery of care, and educational and other innovations in the structures of work all tend to affect employee-management relations.

In recent years, the country has witnessed a variety of movements toward more equality among groups. Pressures and legal decisions regarding sexual and racial discrimination highlight this major shift. Minorities and, more recently, women, have worked hard to achieve equal treatment in access to jobs, better and more equitable pay, promotion, and career opportunities. This movement occurs almost simultaneously with the move to establish health care as a right. Simultaneously, an educational level of two years beyond high school approaches a norm for the community, rather than being the exception. These trends can easily be translated into pressures for unions and other devices to further the overall objective.

The growth of trade unions comes mostly from services and white collar groups, with a declining proportion from manufacturing. Limited slowdowns, picketing, and strikes among teachers, firemen, postal workers, and policemen seem acceptable to the community; why not health care organizations as well? Interns, residents, salaried physicians, and, increasingly, private physicians look to unions as an appropriate vehicle for expressing their interests. With this lead, few of the less prestigious professions seem likely to continue to view unions as an inappropriate means of dealing with employers.

Along with the increasing pressures for equity among many health care workers, and the growing success of unions with other public and professional groups, the changing role of government must be considered. Public policy favoring the right to organize and bargain collectively seems well established in industry generally and now in health care. The interstate commerce clause provides the basic constitutional rationale for federal entry into employee-management relations. Also, in institutions where federal funds provide for the goods or services produced, federal policies regarding work conditions often apply. The increasing federalization of the purchase of health services provides leverage to implement federal policy. It seemed inevitable that the federal government would intervene in the employee-labor-management picture at some point in time. Many other local and national trends contribute to any local situation.

Unions and union activity arise from a variety of forces. Generally, the employees engaging in union activity have some commitment to the working-class status already achieved and share common purposes and problems. Nurses, aides, housekeepers, and laboratory workers have common interests, problems, and the expectation that they will continue to work for the types of organizations currently employing them. The likelihood of moving into the higher ranks of management or becoming independent practitioners is virtually nil.

In our culture, public policy approves and protects unionization of health workers. In 1974, the National Labor Relations Act was changed to protect collective bargaining in nonprofit hospitals. Other types of public-interest workers gained wide recognition and attention in the 1960s. Teachers, firemen, hospital workers and, increasingly, nurses, doctors, and others have insisted upon collective bargaining through unions to express their needs as a group. Some communities and types of agencies, of course, have been more receptive, without the need for legal sanctioning, to this type of recognition than others.

Other cultural factors relate to the position of the worker group in the larger society. Minorities in recent years — including women — have worked out some perceived inequities and grievances through union mechanisms.

Specific organizational problems and situations also lead to union organization. Firemen, electricians, and maintenance workers often belong to an established union that insists on representing them wherever they work. The individual in these circumstances promotes his own potential mobility within the craft by maintaining his position in the union.

In addition to the factors that give rise to unionism, a variety of elements, including individual factors such as age, sex, family background, race, and religion, influence decisions to join and participate. The desire for improved working conditions, in terms of physical factors, management policies, and supervision influence individual and group decisions. Economic gains in overall wage levels and equitable structures within the work group and industry play a major role. Personal goals for participation, leadership, upward mobility, and "the good life" in general also enter into the decision to join. Like physicians in private practice, employees in the industry wish to have some control over the work they do and the conditions surrounding it. Employees and many employers find that unions assist in establishing a semijudicial method for handling grievances, a process difficult to implement successfully when workers must operate as individuals in the give-and-take associated with this situation.

From the standpoint of the unions, organizing serves several purposes. Wages within the industry can be stabilized more easily and equitably if all of the same types of workers are unionized and paying dues. More members and larger dues bases provide power for the union and its leaders, both in the community and within the larger structure of union organizations. Personal and organizational ideologies also play a part. Many union people believe that workers can achieve equity, fairness, and a proper place in work only if they organize into unions.

POST-TEST 8–3

The registered nurses in the hospital have asked for union representation and collective bargaining.

1. What are some of the changes in our society that may be influential in this decision?

2. Why would the nurses' association seek to unionize nurses?

3. What are some of the personal and organizational factors that might influence individual decisions?

ELEMENTS OF A POSITIVE EMPLOYEE-MANAGEMENT RELATIONS PROGRAM

In developing your own positive approach to employee relations, keep in mind the fact that work relations should produce positive outcomes, both for the organization and for those employed to do work on its behalf. The basic systems model suggests consideration of the elements depicted in Figure 19.

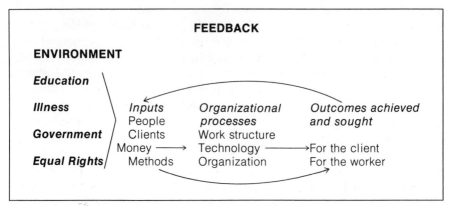

Figure 19   Components of employee-management relations.

Sensitivity to the Environment

This model suggests that the environment affects the inputs to the organization, which in turn has an impact upon the way work proceeds,
leading to some further impact upon outcomes. Management can achieve
a variety of organizational goals by changing the combinations of inputs
and many of the ways in which work becomes organized and is performed. The organization may also be modified by environmental pressures. This model can also be applied to any level of organization to further understand what should be changed in order to achieve
organizational and individual goals.

Sensitivity to the Inputs of the System

Consider the problem of determining pay for a group of clerical employees. One could consider the inputs (young, unmarried women) and
the quality of work as given factors, leaving the only variable the manner
in which rewards are given. The systems model suggests other possible intervention points. First, one could modify the types of persons recruited.
Go to older persons primarily, or perhaps work with school counselors to
obtain referrals for girls with either short-term work interest or with career interest. It might be feasible to recruit also for candidates with aptitude and then offer training yourself.

Alternatively, the secretarial pool could be reorganized around a system whereby senior career employees work with several younger, shorter-
term employees, thus differentiating the roles and allowing for experience
and seniority to have greater meaning in terms of assignment and pay; or
one could contract with a typing service, thus shifting to a third party the
problem of how to organize and produce.

The systems model, when applied to various organizational levels, often suggests solution areas outside the immediate problem area. Whatever level one chooses as the most appropriate for crafting a solution, a number of concerns must still be given attention.

Positive Relationships with Supervisors

Employee attitudes and performance depend heavily upon the employees' relationship with supervisors. Giving credit, encouraging initiative and growth, giving reasons with instructions, providing opportunities for the ventilation of feelings, and being willing to accept responsibility all stand out as indicators of effective supervision. Administration needs to encourage and actively develop communication downward, upward, and across the organization. Support by administration for supervisors and assistance in becoming more effective constitute key ingredients in a program of employee-management relations.

Every manager should know and understand the facts about every employee's background, education, family, and aspirations. Attitudes about work satisfaction, work history, and general work record all represent factors that will influence behavior and must be considered in making decisions about an individual and a work situation.

Realistic Goals

To achieve satisfaction from work, employees need goals that can be achieved, supervisory assistance, job knowledge, good working conditions, significant work, and compensation that represents equity in terms of contribution and relative position in the organization and the community. Supervisors set the tone for interpersonal relations and should be careful to analyze before acting, avoid favoritism, and remain positive in all of their relations.

Equity

At the work level, fairness and equity stand out as hallmarks of good relations. Good communication, counseling and coaching for individuals, and sound work training also provide the basis for effective relationships and superior work performance. Supporting these attributes, the organization needs to be up-to-date in its personnel policies and practices, with professional people managing these concerns.

POST-TEST 8–4

State five elements of a positive employee-management relations program.

SUMMARY

Sound employee relations require careful attention to the basic condition of work: namely, that exchange and equity constitute the basis for the written or unwritten relationship. Environmental forces beyond the control of an individual organization set the tone for internal relations but still leave the manager in a position to make a variety of changes to accommodate without sacrificing institutional goals for excellence in the delivery of health services. Unions reflect certain cultural norms and represent an organized method by which employees may choose to achieve equity and advancement of their interest.

By viewing the organization and work unit as a system, the manager opens up a variety of possibilities to find and implement more effective programs.

RECAP EXERCISE 8

Mr. Collins, hospital administrator, just received word that a delegation of employees wishes to see him about some employee concerns regarding wages, working conditions, and employee morale. Research Hospital serves as one of three major teaching hospitals for Cure Medical School, which is located in a major metropolitan area where the population has shifted over the years from being primarily white upper and middle class to one that is mostly poor and unemployed or marginally employed, with over 60 per cent black people.

The head of the delegation is Ms. Turner, a 30-year-old black woman who worked as a nursing aide for five years before completing a surgical technician program. She now works primarily with several leading surgeons on highly specialized procedures. Another member of the delegation is Michael Murphy, a second-year resident in pediatrics. George Dunn, a black man, represents the housekeeping area. Mr. Dunn is 54 years old and has 20 years of service with the hospital. Shirley Jones, a 23-year-old nurse with a master's degree in public health nursing, runs an outreach center funded by the office of Economic Opportunity in the neighborhood to serve ambulatory patients. Other workers not named will represent the nursing, dietary, and maintenance departments.

Mr. Collins realizes that the meeting may be somewhat tense, since delegations of this sort are unusual. The hospital has recently completed a wage and salary survey but has not yet implemented the recommendations. In spite of his ability to know of most of the problem areas within the institution, Mr. Collins does not wish to try to respond immediately to specific grievances without more detailed investigation. However, he does not wish to come to the meeting without being able to at least review some of the principles of sound employee relations and to exchange opinions with the group.

In light of the material presented in this chapter and preceding chapters, what key principles would you suggest that Mr. Collins review and be prepared to discuss at the meeting?

REFERENCES

1. Aspen Systems Corporation: *Health Care Labor Manual.* Washington, D.C., Aspen Systems Corporation, 1974.
2. Clark, Grover: The unionization of hospital professionals. *Personnel* 40–46, July–August, 1970.
3. *Employers' Labor Relations Guidebook.* Indianapolis, Indiana State Chamber of Commerce, 1970.
4. Herzberg, Frederick: *Work and the Nature of Man.* Cleveland, World Publishing Co., 1966.
5. Metzger, Norman, and Poiter, Dennis D.: *Labor-Management Relations in the Health Services Industry.* Washington, D.C., Science and Health Publications, Inc., 1972.
6. Rothman, William: *A Bibliography of Collective Bargaining in Hospitals and Related Facilities, 1959–1968.* Ann Arbor, Institute of Labor and Industrial Relations, 1970.
7. Schoderbek, Peter, and Reif, W. E.: *Job Enlargement: Key to Improved Performance.* Ann Arbor, University of Michigan Press, 1969.
8. Sloane, Arthur, and Whitney, Fred: *Labor Relations,* 2nd ed., Englewood Cliffs, N. J., Prentice-Hall, Inc., 1971.
9. Steenfield, J.: Health manpower—dilemma or solvable problems? In *Health Manpower Dilemma.* New York, National League for Nursing, 1970.
10. Walton, Richard E.: *Interpersonal Peacemaking: Confrontations and Third Party Consultation* Reading, Mass., Addison-Wesley Publishing Co., 1969.
11. Yoder, D.: *Personnel Management and Industrial Relations.* Englewood Cliffs, N. J., Prentice-Hall, Inc., 1970.

Selected Readings

INTRODUCTION

The effective manager must seek cost-saving alternatives in solving institutional problems. There are many creative and routine methods for coming to grips with tough issues and difficult problems. This process is partly one of finding feasible alternatives and working out methods for implementing decisions. It also depends increasingly upon well-educated and well-trained personnel who are motivated to achieve both individual and institutional goals. McCool speaks directly to the issues related to viewing and using the hospitals and health service systems as educational/learning systems. Match et al. address a more current but equally important issue, namely, operating effectively with collective bargaining, a recent requirement under federal law. Unions, shop stewards, formal grievance systems, and even strikes now exist and must be understood by the health administrator.

Health care institutions must continually make decisions and solve problems. As the industry grows more complex and faces rapid changes in technology and delivery of care, it is essential to have properly prepared and educated personnel whose human and economic needs are met. McCool lays out a total systems model for considering the hospital as an educational system. Such models, as suggested in the earlier modules relating to conceptual skills, help decision makers to consider all of the aspects of problems in establishing, conducting, and evaluating educational programs.

Exercises

Consider the educational programs associated with your own area of responsibility.
1. Do they fit with the goals of individuals?
2. Do they fit with the needs of the organization and its clients?
3. Are they organized in a cost-effective fashion?
4. Are they shared with others?
5. Are they evaluated properly in terms of quality and cost?

Many of the factors associated with unions are described in the article by Match et al. and in Learning Module 8. It seems likely that a much larger portion of the industry will be organized by unions in the future. Professional nurses and physicians, most notably house staff, already have union contracts and have struck in a number of locations. Attending physicians and salaried physicians have used collective bargaining and other forms of collective action to gain power over those whose actions were formerly difficult to direct.

Exercises

1. What are the probably directions of union organizing at your own institution?
2. Are there situations in your area which, if modified or tackled systematically, might lead to a decision that would promote the interest of the institution and the people employed by the organization?
3. Are there steps you might take to improve the climate of work in your own unit?

   (*Note:* While these questions and the answers to them might have the effect of lessening the changes caused by union organization, they will also constitute a necessary part of working effectively with organized groups of employees.)

Unionization, Strikes, Threatened Strikes, and Hospitals — The View from Hospital Management

ROBERT K. MATCH, ARNOLD H. GOLDSTEIN, AND HAROLD L. LIGHT

The history of union organizing efforts in the hospital field is discussed in this article, along with the factors judged necessary for successful union organizing. The role played by labor legislation in the unionization of hospital workers is shown, and the influences of the National Labor Relations Act, the Taft-Hartley amendments, and labor legislation at the local level are described.

Management has largely resisted unionization because of the social nature of hospitals. Competitive market forces do not confront the not-for-profit hospitals, which are dependent upon third-party reimbursement. While strikes are an integral and essential part of collective bargaining in industry, they are, in fact, detrimental to hospitals because of these institutions' concern with human life. Despite laws and assurances from labor leaders that strikes will not occur, strikes have been used as a method for resolving disputes, though they are basically inconsistent with the economic characteristics and objectives of the hospital.

The authors conclude that arbitration awards should be made by arbitrators appointed from outside of the local region of the hospital involved, and that, because of the catastrophic effect of strikes upon patients as well as employees, arbitration awards should be required, should be binding upon both parties, and should be federally enforced.

THE DEVELOPMENT OF UNIONS IN HOSPITALS

Although the first hospital employee union was recognized more than 50 years ago, there were only scattered instances of collective bargaining in hospitals prior to the 1960s. Recently, however, hospital administrators and trustees have expressed concern over the rapid increase of unionization of hospital employees. Their concern has been motivated by the extent of collective bargaining activities, the rate of union expansion, the number and effects of work stoppages, and the impact of unionization upon the hospital's ability to function and on the management of its finances and resources.

Int. J. Health Services 5:27–36, 1975. Copyright©1975, Baywood Publishing Co.

Historically, union organizing efforts and the recognition of unions have moved at a rather slow pace. The recent rapid growth of unions in all segments of the hospital work force is attributed to many factors. These include a national drive to organize hospital workers mounted by various unions throughout the United States in 1959, the inadequacy of hospital management policies regarding personnel, including policies on wages and increments, the lack of grievance machinery and of proper supervision, the general absence of effective employee communication and participation, and the economic and political forces that have shaped the financing of health services in the 1970s.

Labor's position was expressed by Nelson H. Cruikshank, Director of the Department of Social Security of the AFL-CIO, in the July 1959 issue of *The Modern Hospital* (1):

> Organized labor often speaks of "democracy in the workplace." To its millions of members, this phrase can be translated to mean a voice in working conditions and a sense of human dignity and respect on the job.... It is hard to believe that any carefully considered "principle" can serve to deny these hospital employees the same rights presently enjoyed by millions of other American workers.

Unionism has, in effect, provided the employee with a voice in the determination of wages, hours, and personnel practices. It has also provided the employee with a sense of security and strength in numbers, and has helped employees feel that there is a skilled organization to represent them.

In an article entitled "Nation's Hospitals Face Union Drive," in the same issue of *The Modern Hospital,* an additional factor in labor's organizing efforts in the hospitals was noted (2):

> Many observers believed the nation's top union leaders had become alarmed because membership in the huge industrial unions had been declining in recent years, with a resulting loss in union revenues. "The hospital working force is a rich, new source of dues-paying union members, if it can be developed," an industrialist told a group of hospital administrators at one of the 1959 hospital conventions.

Unions are always seeking new members; the labor force has doubled from 40 million, 35 years ago, to some 88 million today, and the size of the increased labor pool is viewed by unions as a fresh resource for their organizing efforts. They feel that they should organize the unorganized in all areas, but especially view the health care industry as fertile territory for their efforts because it may conceivably become the largest single employer among the industries of the United States. Competition among unions for members from the hospitals also exists. Thus, the Garment Workers, Meat Packers, Teamsters, the Service Workers International Union, the American Federation of State, County and Municipal Employees, the Communications Workers of

America, the National Union of Hospital and Health Care Employees, and others all have organized hospital workers (3).

Minority groups have also become more militant and involved and have recognized collective bargaining as a method for equalizing relationships.

The pathway to unionization in the hospital field started basically with federal employees, progressed to state, municipal, and proprietary employees, and finally reached those in the nonprofit sector, the only sector previously exempt from labor laws, except in states which had passed such legislation. Because recent amendments to the Taft-Hartley Law have now removed this exemption, a huge potential membership pool has been opened, in the labor-intensive, not-for-profit health care facilities. These facilities employ an estimated 1.5 million workers, only 12 per cent of whom are now unionized.

Once the national campaign to organize hospital workers was mounted, the unions concentrated their efforts mainly on nonprofessional workers, whose wages and working conditions were totally inadequate. For example, in 1959, the lowest hiring scale for unskilled workers in a hospital in New York City was $147 a month or approximately $35 per week (4). It is important to point out, however, that even while employees were receiving such low wages, some voluntary hospitals in New York City were incurring operating deficits. These deficits came about because sources of support for patient services did not provide adequate reimbursement to the institutions and because the great advances made in medical technology required more expensive equipment and skilled personnel. There is no doubt that hospital workers were in essence bearing the burden of the inadequate financing and were in fact subsidizing hospital operations.

While present patterns of formal bargaining are partly a function of hospital size, the distribution of union recognition by region illustrates that other forces also are involved. One important factor has been the laws regulating labor relations. The National Labor Relations Act (Wagner Act) was one such law. Passed in 1935, it did not specifically exclude nonprofit hospitals, and, in 1944, a Federal Court affirmed the National Labor Relations Board's jurisdiction over hospitals (5). However, in 1947, the Taft-Hartley amendments to the federal law excluded from its coverage corporations or associations operating a hospital, if no part of the net earnings inured to the benefit of any private shareholder or individual (6). In 1967, the National Labor Relations Board asserted jurisdiction over proprietary hospitals and nursing homes even though the Board had, historically, refused such jurisdiction.

In reversing its former position, the Board found that proprietary hospitals with gross revenues of $250,000 would, in fact, affect interstate commerce because skilled personnel were obtained from outside the local area, and such hospitals were no longer charitable because of the presence of the third-party payors. A mechanism was also provided to prevent recognition strikes, with the Board stating that hospital employees should have the same rights to collective bargaining as others. In addition, the Board ruled that nursing homes operated in a similar fashion to proprietary hospitals and so accepted jurisdiction over facilities that received annual gross revenues of $100,000 or more (7).

Several states also enacted their own labor relations laws. In each of ten states, nongovernmental nonprofit hospitals are now included under the provisions of the statue, which generally requires collective bargaining recognition.

What happened in federal hospitals is an example of this regulatory influence. The unusual level of collective bargaining in federal hospitals since 1967 can be attributed almost entirely to an executive order issued five years earlier. Prior to 1962, federal employees did not have the right to bargain collectively, but an executive order issued in that year by President John F. Kennedy established collective bargaining rights for federal employees, including those in federal hospitals.

An important factor in the increase of collective bargaining in hospitals has been the extent of collective bargaining generally in an area. If a large part of the area's work force is unionized, hospital employees in that area are prone to organize in order to obtain additional income or benefits. It is probable that the public response to unions is more favorable in such areas than in areas of low union membership.

The American Hospital Association surveyed the extent of collective bargaining in hospitals in 1961, 1967, and 1970 (8). Findings from the 1970 study clearly indicate that the extent and rate of unionization continues to increase (see Table 1). As with other sectors of the economy, union organizing in the hospital sector tends to occur in larger work units. Table 2 indicates that the bed size of hospitals is a factor in explaining both the extent and growth of collective bargaining in hospitals (9).

Table 1   Extent of Collective Bargaining Contracts in Hospitals in 1961, 1967, and 1970 by Control of Hospital

CONTROL	1961		1967		1970	
	TOTAL NUMBER OF REGISTERED HOSPITALS	PERCENTAGE WITH CONTRACTS	TOTAL NUMBER OF REGISTERED HOSPITALS	PERCENTAGE WITH CONTRACTS	TOTAL NUMBER OF REGISTERED HOSPITALS	PERCENTAGE WITH CONTRACTS
All hospitals	6,923	3.0	7,172	7.7	7,123	14.7
Federal	437	0.0	416	22.6	408	52.0
Nonfederal	6.486	3.2	2,141 [sic]	6.8	6,715	12.4
Nongovernmental not-for-profit	3,588	4.3	3,692	8.2	3,600	12.4
For-profit	973	4.3	923	4.9	858	8.0
State and local	1,925	1.0	2,141	5.3	2,257	14.1

[a]Source, reference 8.

Table 2 Extent of Collective Bargaining Contracts and Requests for Collective Bargaining Recognition in Hospitals in 1967 and 1970 by Bed Size and Census Division[a]

CATEGORIZATION	1967			1970		
	TOTAL NUMBER OF REGISTERED HOSPITALS	PERCENTAGE WITH CONTRACTS	PERCENTAGE WITH REQUESTS	TOTAL NUMBER OF REGISTERED HOSPITALS	PERCENTAGE WITH CONTRACTS	PERCENTAGE WITH REQUESTS
All hospitals	7,172	7.7	5.2	7,123	14.7	3.7
Bed size category						
6–24	542	1.3	0.7	447	2.2	0.7
25–49	1,629	2.4	1.0	1,475	4.3	0.7
50–99	1,734	5.4	2.6	1,713	8.5	1.8
100–199	1,365	8.9	5.3	1,473	14.7	3.7
200–299	686	14.0	9.3	698	25.2	5.9
300–399	375	14.7	12.5	427	24.2	7.3
400–499	220	15.5	14.1	261	33.7	9.6
500+	621	17.4	14.7	629	38.6	11.0
Division						
New England	415	5.8	8.7	414	21.7	5.1
Middle Atlantic	896	11.4	7.4	888	25.0	6.3
South Atlantic	925	3.4	4.1	949	7.8	3.1
East North Central	1,169	8.7	8.6	1,132	17.6	6.7
East South Central	551	3.4	2.5	534	5.6	2.1
West North Central	901	9.2	2.7	903	11.3	1.9
West South Central	956	1.4	1.6	940	3.8	0.5
Mountain	441	4.3	4.1	438	8.9	3.9
Pacific	918	17.6	6.3	925	27.5	3.6

[a]Source, reference 8.

ORGANIZATION OF PROFESSIONALS

Employee organization in collective bargaining, while clearly established in the American labor movement, did not directly affect the health professionals until recently when some groups began to concern themselves with the need to organize. Dissatisfaction regarding their own position in relation to insurers, hospitals, and government, and trends in the economy, have been greatly responsible for health professionals beginning to organize.

In 1967, the AFL-CIO Council for Professional, Scientific, and Cultural Employees was established by nine international unions to facilitate the organization of 10 million professional employees in the United States. Special emphasis was placed on organizing employees in the hospital sector (10).

Professional associations are also actively involved in trying to upgrade and negotiate terms and conditions for their memberships. The American Nurses Association (ANA), for instance, has long sought economic protection and other advantages for the nursing professional. In 1937 the ANA recommended that nurses not join unions and suggested that they work to improve their professional situation through the Association. Later the house of delegates of the ANA officially initiated an economic security program and urged that all state and district nurses' associations push this program. . . (11).

By January 1974, 475 contracts had been negotiated by 33 state nurses' associations, covering approximately 65,000 registered nurses and including 381 contracts negotiated in 11 states with labor laws that protect the rights of nurses to enter into collective bargaining units.

As with nonprofessionals, organized labor has also encouraged the organization of professional employees because of the potential membership pool that they offer. Professional employees are now faced with the choice of affiliating with their professional associations or with trade unions. The complicating factor for the professional is the fear that his appropriate interests may not be completely protected in units in which he is greatly outnumbered by nonprofessional employees; in some instances, there is the added philosophical conflict about the ethical propriety of union membership.

The Committee of Interns and Residents, which at present is not formally affiliated within the trade union movement, has had correspondence with George Meany, President of the AFL-CIO, on the subject of unionization. Practicing physicians are interested in influencing the climate in which medicine is practiced as well as the income they receive from it. Complaints have been registered that income has not kept pace with the cost of practicing medicine and that third-party payors are telling physicians how to practice. According to a recent article (12), William L. Kircher, Director of Organization for the AFL-CIO, "has a sympathetic attitude toward the principle of doctors' unionization." However, he does not feel that doctors will be able to use collective bargaining to get a fair economic break from the government and other third parties unless they become employees of those parties.

Mr. Kircher is aware that doctors, in the past, have denounced unions, even though now they are talking about, and actually forming their own union. He understands that they realize there is strength in unionism and their previous feelings about unions could very well be dissipated by what they see as their present unfavorable environment (12).

A recent national survey taken among physicians indicated that three of every five doctors believe they should unionize (12). The survey also found that a number of doctors would be willing to turn to professional labor leaders. Another survey indicated that if they considered it necessary, more than half the doctors responding would strike—provided that emergency services were not interrupted (12).

MANAGEMENT'S VIEW TOWARD UNIONIZATION OF HOSPITAL WORKERS

Hospital trustees and administrators have been deeply concerned about the possible effects of unionization upon already difficult hospi-

tal operations and, with several exceptions, they have opposed the organization of hospital workers. Many questions were posed which
dealt with management's concern as to whether union activities might
so interfere with management that hospital operations would be made
more difficult than they already are. They have argued that charitable
nonprofit hospitals are not a legitimate area for union organizational
efforts because the objectives of these institutions are social rather
than economic (13). Deep concern has been expressed about the possible impact of strikes and slowdowns upon patient care, and such actions have been labeled as irresponsible, since the basic stakes are not
income distribution but human life (13). With increased labor costs, the
already underfinanced not-for-profit hospitals were further inhibited in
expansion of programs and services because of the increased competition for a limited number of dollars. Regardless of the concerns
expressed by management, however, strikes have occurred, employees
in hospitals have been organized, and a new era of collective bargaining in the hospital industry has begun.

COLLECTIVE BARGAINING

According to Davey (14),

> Collective bargaining is defined as a continuing institutional rela-
> tionship between an employer entity and a labor organization represent-
> ing exclusively a defined group of employees concerned with the negoti-
> ation, administration, interpretation and enforcement of written
> agreements covering joint understanding as to wages or salaries, rates of
> pay, hours of work, and other conditions of employment.

In 1959, Ray Amberg, President of the American Hospital Association, wrote of collective bargaining as follows (15):

> Collective bargaining has arisen as a desire for a democratic method
> to solve the problems of employer-employee relations principally due to
> the lack of proper functioning of the direct employer-employee method.
> ... But we no longer possess the right in many cases to deny our workers
> the privilege of collective bargaining provided they feel that the old sys-
> tem is unjust, unfair, or for any other reason not in their best interest.

The problem with collective bargaining in hospitals is that where
strong hospital unions exist it is difficult to accommodate the interests
of employees, payors, patients, and hospitals because of the pressure
that such unions can exert to support their demands. The difference
between nonprofit hospitals and private enterprises is that competitive,
product-market forces do not confront the former. Product-market
forces, in effect, can restrain large settlements at the bargaining table

because of the impact they could have on sales and competitions, which could possibly result in unemployment. Such market restrictions do not apply as directly to the not-for-profit hospitals, where the vast portion of hospital operating revenue depends on third-party payors which, in essence, means that organized consumers and intermediaries can participate in decisions that pertain to the organization, delivery, and cost of health services. . . .

Confronting the hospital are present and potential constraints on the use of the cost pass-through mechanism. These constraints are political forces, rather than product-market forces; they are reflected in the increasing role of governmental and quasi-governmental agencies in the hospital managerial function. Furthermore, without product-market forces to limit hospital cost increases, payors will have to protect their economic interest through direct participation in the hospital managerial function and by lobbying for government regulatory control. In either case, the absence of market forces makes hospital collective bargaining a multiparty process, in contrast to the traditional bipartite character of private enterprise collective bargaining. In industries that are dependent upon government subsidies for continued operation or in which product-market forces are evaluated as not protecting the so-called "public interest," the multiparty character of collective bargaining is increasingly evident. . . .

The growing of number of internal and external participants in the hospital managerial function raises a critical question: with whom should hospital unions negotiate? In an institution with strong employee organizations and regulated hospital income, hospital management is a middleman in the bargaining that takes place between those who finance hospital care and the employees who provide the services. For example, negotiations between the League of Voluntary Hospitals, New York City, and Local 1199 are fundamentally between state officials and powerful union. An accord must be struck between increasing payroll costs and increasing insurance premiums and subsidies. . . .

A recurrent theme in the literature on hospital collective bargaining is that strikes result primarily from the lack of alternate methods to resolve the issue of representation. This premise concludes that, should hospital employees be accorded representation election rights, the occurrence of work stoppages would be minimized. The record of the past decade does not fully support such a conclusion. Strike activity during the 1950s and in the mid-1960s was primarily organizational. During the past five years, however, an increasing number of legal and illegal work stoppages have resulted from bargaining impasses.

STRIKES

Strikes have often been used as a weapon to resolve labor disputes. In private industry, most conflicts which arise in the formulation of a new contract may be resolved by a test of bargaining power, including the use of the strike. This test is deemed an essential ingredient of the collective bargaining process. But disputes in industry rarely have an impact on life and death. In the health care sector, when patient care and welfare is jeopardized, there has been ample demonstration that even where it has been specifically illegal for hospital employees to strike, the strike weapon has been used. An example of this is the series of strikes by District 1199 against hospitals in New York. Labor leaders have contended that as labor-management relationships in the hospital industry mature, there will be fewer strikes.

Strikes against the voluntary hospitals in New York City have been, perhaps by far, the most critical and publicized labor disputes in the entire hospital industry; these have occurred in violation of pledges not to strike made by the union, and have continued even after the courts have ordered the strikers to return to work.

An official of District 1199 of the National Union of Hospital and Health Care Employees had indicated that "it was never their aim to make a strike 100 per cent effective. They wanted a strike to be effective enough to make a hospital capitulate rather than evacuate (17)." Another official of District 1199 was also quoted as saying that strikes were a thing of the past in New York State: "Now that all of the state is covered by progressive hospital labor law," he said, "the days of hospital strikes in the state are over—unqualifiedly (17)."

Yet, in spite of these previous no-strike assurances, in 1973 the 48 member hospitals of the League of Voluntary Homes and Hospitals in New York City (which accounted for about half of the hospital beds in the city) were crippled by an eight-day strike by 30,000 District 1199 employees that severely curtailed the services at these hospitals and nursing homes.

This strike resulted from the Cost of Living Council's failure to come to a decision on a 7.5 per cent pay and benefit increase. The strike continued in the face of a $500,000 fine to the union, and a personal fine to its officers, and even after the City's Health Department had declared a state of emergency.

The League of Voluntary Homes and Hospitals estimated that 12,000 of the 23,000 beds at the 48 institutions were emptied as patients were discharged or transferred to other institutions. During the strike, hospitals shut down all outpatient clinics and permitted only emergency admissions. At least two hospitals closed services entirely. Pickets prevented garbage pick-up, and at 43 institutions the accumulated waste was declared a fire and health hazard. Acts of violence at the picket line occurred, with as many as 22 persons arrested in a single day.

As Miller (18) has pointed out, the right to strike generally given to employees in private industry has not been readily given to hospital employees because it has been amply demonstrated that work stoppages have an impact on the availability of patient services. The threat of strike and the strike itself in the health care sector provide a disproportionate amount of coercive power that can be placed in the hands of a strong union.

Miller believes that, as a method of resolving disputes, the strike is basically inconsistent with both the economic characteristics and the service objectives of hospitals. The consequences of nonagreement between a strongly organized union and a hospital fall primarily upon the public. Miller (18) continues by stating that:

> The ability of the hospital and striking employees to endure economic losses is not relevant in the manner that is normally associated with the costs of work stoppages in private enterprise . . . . In private enterprise, a strike performs its function of inducing concessions from both union and management if the employees and the firm suffer economic losses and if the primary impact of the strike is upon the employees and the firm. For an increasing number of private sector industries, as for not-for-profit hospitals political tolerance of the strike becomes a relevant question when the primary and immediate impact of the strike is upon third-party or public interests. Political considerations relate both to disruptions in the availability of essential services and to the impact of negotiations upon patient charges. Tactics for manipulating political intervention are integral elements in the use or threat of legal and illegal work stoppages. Indeed, it has not been uncommon for hospitals to take a firm position in negotiations, with the intent of placing responsibility upon the government and the union for subsequent cost increases . . . . Whether union participation without the strike is meaningful largely depends upon the degree to which substitute procedures are acceptable to the various parties of direct interest.

ALTERNATIVES

There are several alternatives to the strike in the process of collective bargaining. These include fact-finding, voluntary arbitration, and compulsory arbitration. With the exception of compulsory arbitration, these alternatives are largely dependent upon the agreement of both parties. Fact finding is not binding upon the parties and both have the right to accept or reject the recommendations. In the use of voluntary arbitration, both the union and management can start the process, determine the issues, and select the panel. Compulsory arbitration, in the view of some experts, is detrimental to the bargaining process because both parties have no choice in the matter. The effect of compulsory arbitration in the Minneapolis-St. Paul area was noted as follows:

> In contrast to New York City, the availability of compulsory arbitration procedures has shaped contractual provisions in Minneapolis-St. Paul. During the past 22 years contracts between Local 113 (Hospital and Institutional Employees Union) and the Twin City Hospital Association have been determined in large measure through compulsory arbitration.

The dependence of Local 113 and the hospital association upon arbitration of new contract terms is one result of a poor working relationship between the two parties. Their contracts have been a cumbersome accumulation of arbitrated provisions. The parties have had little success in clarifying the agreements through direct negotiations and have come to accept new contract arbitration as standard practice. These deficiencies notwithstanding, the hospitals have been essentially free of work stoppages.

Experience in the San Francisco Bay area would suggest that extensive influence by third-party interests upon union-hospital negotiations can be an important element for stable collective bargaining under voluntary arbitration. During the 1940s, the San Francisco City Labor Council was largely responsible for bringing about recognition of Local 250 (Hospital and Institutional Workers Union) by San Francisco hospitals, and the Council has since influenced the conduct of hospital collective bargaining. However, militants within the Local have charged that the Council's concern with charges and services restrains economic gains that could be accomplished with greater coercive pressures applied by the union. The aggressiveness of the California State Nurses Association, which was involved in a lengthy strike in the San Francisco Bay area in 1974, may have undermined the apparent stability of collective bargaining enjoyed by all parties concerned.

CONCLUSION

Hospital unions have derived great benefits from the arbitration process because of both the way in which arbitration panels have been selected and the influence of local and state politicians upon settlements which have traditionally been supported through the mechanism of cost-pass-throughs. Confronted by new union contracts, inflationary contract settlements, and regulatory confinements, and confounded in their attempts to regulate cost increases because of fear of government control reprisals, increasingly hospitals have had to scrape for their economic viability. Many such institutions are bankrupt or on the verge of bankruptcy. While hospital management would like to see employee wages determined with reference to both economics and patient care, the collective bargaining process at the local level has not always been satisfactory to the hospital's position. Arbitration awards should be made by arbitrators who have no local vested interest in the settlement. Accordingly, arbitrators should be appointed from outside of the local region. Because of the catastrophic nature of strikes upon the care and welfare of patients, as well as upon employees, the arbitration award should be binding upon both parties and should be federally enforced.

REFERENCES

1. Cruikshank, N. H. The case for the unionization of hospital workers. *Mod. Hosp.* 93(1):71–72, 1959.
2. Nation's hospitals face union drive. *Mod. Hosp.* 93(1):61–62, 1959.
3. *A Directory of Public Employees Organizations. A Guide to the Major Organizations Representing State and Local Public Employees*, p. 44. U.S. Department of Labor, Labor Management Service Administration, November 1971.
4. Cherkasky, M. Why we signed a union agreement. *Mod. Hosp.* 93:64–70, July 1959.
5. Central Dispensary and Emergency Hospital. U NLRB, S7 NLRB 393, aff'd F. 2d 853 (D.C. Circ. 1944).
6. Labor Management Relations Act, 1947, 61 stat., 136, 29, U.S.C. ch. 141 sec. 2(2).
7. Graham, H. E. Effects on NLRB jurisdictional charge on union organizing activity in the proprietary health care sector, p. 278. In *Proceedings of the 24th Annual Winter Meeting, December 27–28, 1971.* Industrial Relations Research Association, 1972.
8. AHA research capsules No. 6. *Hospitals* 46:217–218, April 1972.
9. Miller, J. D., and Shurtell, S. M. Hospital unionization: A study of the trends. *Hospitals* 43(16):67–73, 1969.
10. Pointer, D. D., and Cannedy, L. L. Organizing of professionals. *Hospitals* 46(6):70–73, 1972.
11. Munger, M. D. American nurses program to promote collective bargaining. *Hospital Topics* p. 21, May 1974.
12. Urlich, S. Will your appendectomy be performed by a member of the AFL–CIO? *Mod. Hosp.* 121(4): 63–67, 1973.
13. Remarks outlining the New York voluntary hospitals' position with regard to unions and threats of strikes given by Martin R. Steinberg, M.D., Director, Mount Sinai Hospital, at a meeting of voluntary hospital representatives requested by New York Commissioner of Labor Felix, April 16, 1959.
14. Davey, H. S. *Contemporary Collective Bargaining*, Ed. 3, p. 3. Prentice-Hall, New York, 1972.
15. Amberg, R. Your president reports (editorial). *Hospitals* 33(11): 51, 1959.
16. Miller, R. L. The hospital-union relationship, part 1. *Hospitals* 45(9):49–54, 1971.
17. Carlson, D. R. Labor union: Color it white, black, or red. *Mod. Hosp.* 105(2):107–111, 1965.
18. Miller, R. L. The hospital-union relationship, part 2. *Hospitals* 45(10):52–56, 1971.

The Hospital: An Educational System

Barbara P. McCool, PhD

Demands for education within the hospital have multiplied, and administrators are becoming more concerned about the organization, financing, and evaluation of educational programs and their long-range impact on patient care. Several simultaneously converging forces have caused this increased emphasis on learning. The knowledge explosion has precipitated such a proliferation of information about improved treatment modalities and health delivery mechanisms that professionals must attend lectures, short-term courses, and institutes in order to keep abreast. The increased emphasis on quality care through competent manpower has caused licensing and professional groups to stress continuing education as a condition of relicensure. Recent court decisions which have made the hospital responsible for the practice of medicine have forced administrators to reevaluate the skill and competence of their personnel. Finally, self-actualization and life-long learning have become the goals of many individuals. In response to this phenomenon, educational institutions have made instruction more individualized and self-paced.

Medical and nursing education always have been important objectives for hospitals. Large medical centers have served as clinical laboratories for student physicians, nurses, and allied health professionals, while community hospitals have offered internships and residencies to young physicians. The nursing departments of most hospitals have sponsored orientation, skill training, continuing education, and management development for their staffs. Recently, however, the educational function of many hospitals has broadened to include all hospital personnel, boards of trustees, patients, and community groups.

As the pressures for educational programming increase, administrators are beset with questions about cost effectiveness, coordination of effort, appropriate use of educational resources, and a host of other related issues. But too often the issues are discussed ad nauseam and in too simplistic a manner; motivation for change is stifled by existing organizational structures; and new system designs fail because individuals are unprepared to implement them.

Boards, administrators, third-party reimbursement agencies, and others concerned with both the quality and cost of care should regard recent enthusiasm for more education skeptically. They should ques-

*Hosp. Progr., 56:*67–71, July, 1975.

tion for what outcome more education is intended. With what type of organizational change or innovation will such education correlate? Will criteria be established to measure the achievement of its goals? Are the most cost effective teaching mechanisms being employed? Do the teachers have the proper credentials and expertise? Does the program represent merely a faddish repackaging of shopworn precepts?

If health care professionals intend to do more than moralize and temporize about more effective education, they must begin to think about ways to evaluate what they have done already to further the complex and diverse hospital educational effort. Education within the hospital setting must be integrated into an over-all system, and an organizational unit must be developed to deliver this service. Only by viewing the hospital's educational role more comprehensively can administrators deal more effectively with educational demand.

This article analyzes the hospital as an educational system. It describes the programs offered by that system and reviews such system components as appropriateness, organization, cost, and effectiveness. The leadership of the hospital must understand the structure of the whole educational function in order to guarantee that quality programs are established for health manpower, consumers, and boards of trustees.

TYPES OF EDUCATIONAL PROGRAMS

Health Manpower. Health manpower programs include preparatory education, inservice education, continuing education, and graduate medical education. Preparatory education, which includes medical, nursing, dental, and allied health professional programs, prepares individuals for initial professional employment in hospitals and other health care agencies. Universities and colleges assume the major responsibility for such preparation; the hospital serves only as a laboratory. The programs are supervised directly by the university faculty, and usually they are financed with federal and state subsidies and tuition payments.

Inservice education, which includes orientation, job skill development, and career mobility programs, helps employees function effectively within a particular hospital setting. Usually these programs are coordinated by a director of education assisted by department heads. Generally they are financed with operating revenues, but a few programs such as nurse's aide or ward clerk training are eligible for government grants.

Continuing education programs help health professionals maintain and improve their specialized knowledge and skills. These programs can be conducted within the hospital, developed cooperatively with universities and professional organizations, or carried on outside the hospital. Financing differs in each case. Often the hospital reimburses the individual by continuing his salary or rebating his tuition.

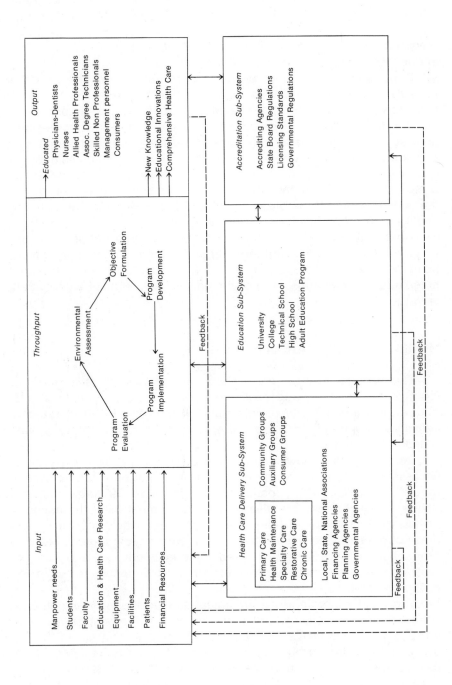

Graduate medical education refers to specialized internship and residency programs based in academic medical centers or hospitals affiliated with a medical school. The programs are supervised by physician coordinators of medical education and financed by grants, endowments, and patient care revenues.

Consumers. Consumer education programs meet the needs of patients who want to know more about their treatment protocol and citizens who are curious about health practices and the factors affecting the delivery system. The patient education programs increasingly are becoming a necessary element of total treatment, and as a result they are financed with operating revenues. The programs designed for members of the community are conducted by a variety of hospital-based professionals, financed by a variety of mechanisms, and serve to inform the consumer about the organization and financing of health care and about his own health status.

Boards of Trustees. Education for the policy maker stresses pertinent information about the legal, organizational, financial, and manpower issues of health care management. This information is disseminated at board meetings, during seminars, or by means of independent study.

MODEL OF THE EDUCATIONAL SYSTEM

The hospital educational system can be viewed as a series of input, transformation, and output factors which synchronize to produce educational programs. This system interacts with the health care delivery, education, and accreditation subsystems. The model is illustrated in the **Figure.**

Input Factors. Input factors are the human and capital resources necessary for a system's operation. The hospital educational system requires students, faculty, patients, equipment, space, and money. Of course, student needs are diverse. Programs must meet the needs of physicians who want to learn the latest diagnostic procedures and those of nurse's aide trainees who must learn a technique as basic as proper bed making. Patients have educational needs, but they also collaborate with the faculty to provide learning experiences for neophyte health professionals.

The faculty is comprised of clinical specialists, professional educators, department heads, and staff members. If the hospital's educational effort is extensive, the faculty is large and centralized in one department. In consortium efforts, the faculty may be responsible for classes in several institutions. Or, if the hospital's effort is more narrow in scope, individuals based in various hospital departments can teach occasional classes.

Physical facilities, space, and money are capital resources. Space is necessary to provide room for instruction, staff offices, and equipment. Facilities should meet present requirements but be flexible enough to accommodate new systems, procedures, teaching machines, and audio-visual materials. Money is needed to hire manpower and provide support services.

Transformation Factors. These activities convert the raw materials (human and capital resources) into a finished product. Transformation is the development and evaluation of educational programs by means of environmental assessment, objective formulation, program planning, implementation, and evaluation.

During environmental assessment, employee educational needs and operating problems are determined. The information collected during surveys, interviews, skill inventories, and observation becomes the basis of educational program objectives.

The objectives in turn become the basis for instructional strategies and program content. Furthermore, well-written objectives which clearly identify desired student behavior will facilitate program evaluation.

Program development refers to the process of defining the content of the educational program, instructional methods, teaching aides, and evaluation procedures to be used. It is the guide by which the program objectives are attained.

Program implementation is the actual administration of the educational program. Prior to implementation, obstacles that may impede the completion of the program should be identified, and student reaction to the program should be sought.

Program evaluation refers to the instructor's, the participant's, his supervisor's, and the patient's assessment of the value of an educational activity. Evaluation is done to determine if the objectives were met and if the program should be repeated, altered, or terminated.

Output Factors. Output factors relate to the products of the system, i.e., skilled health professionals and informed consumers and board members, in addition to innovations in instruction and improved patient care.

Subsystem Interaction. The health care delivery subsystem interacts with the hospital educational system by demanding qualified manpower to delivery primary, specialty, restorative, and chronic care and foster health maintenance. Through the continual updating of manpower skills and knowledge, the delivery system is able to respond to the pressures placed on it for better ways of providing comprehensive, accessible, quality care.

The education subsystem encompasses all of the institutions mandated by society to provide formal educational programs. These include universities, colleges, and technical and vocational schools in addition to primary and secondary schools. All of these institutions are resources for potential manpower and education for the hospital.

Universities, colleges, and technical institutions work directly with hospitals in various ways. During preparatory education, these institutions use the clinical facilities of the hospital to train their student physicians, nurses, therapists, and managers. College-hospital interaction also occurs when the college offers formal courses for certain hospital employee groups. Frequently, continuing adult education programs based in high schools are a collaborative effort between the school and hospital professionals to provide health-related courses.

Accrediting and licensing agencies frequently interact with the hospital educational system. The Joint Commission on Accreditation of Hospitals has specified that boards of trustees are responsible for providing educational programs for every department of the hospital. State boards representing a variety of professional groups require that hospitals request registration identification when hiring professionals. Agencies accrediting health-related educational programs require hospitals to maintain certain physical and manpower standards. Finally, professional groups such as medical societies are requesting that the hospital participate in educational programs for their members.

MANAGEMENT CONSIDERATIONS

An analysis of the hospital educational system using input, transformation, and output factors as well as subsystem relationships is incomplete if specific questions about the management of the educational function within a particular institution are ignored. How can the individual administrator define, organize, finance, and evaluate educational function for his particular institution? The following guidelines can be used when addressing this question.

Premise 1: The definition of the educational function should be congruent with the goals of the hospital.

When selecting educational programs, the administrator should examine the hospital's resources and goals. Because one of the main objectives of any hospital is to provide quality patient care, educational programs always should further this goal. The administrator also should examine the hospital's input and transformation components to determine what programs realistically can be implemented. If the students using the hospital are employees and consumer groups, resources such as faculty, equipment, and space should be selected according to their needs. On the other hand, if the hospital is an academic medical center, the design and evaluation of the clinical programs should meet the needs of a much more sophisticated student population. The objectives and input components of an academic medical center differ from those of a general community hospital. The resources needed for the planning and implementation of programs in the former environment would far surpass those needed in the latter.

Goal congruence also implies that a hospital should do what it does best, i.e., care for patients and look to educational institutions for guidance in the educational function. If the administrator regards the educational subsystem as a necessary part of the hospital's educational system, several possibilities materialize. Educational programs requiring heavy emphasis on didactic learning become the domain of the academic institution while the hospital provides clinical experience. Likewise, the school system can contract with the hospital to provide courses for its employees either at the hospital or in a school near the hospital.

Premise 2: Centralized management and cost sharing should be encouraged when organizing the educational function.

In order to prevent duplication of effort and costly equipment, a director of education should be responsible for the coordination and cost effectiveness of all the educational programs in the hospital. Employees of the department of education should be specialists in the educational process who assist the hospital staff in needs assessment and program planning, implementation, and evaluation. A centralized effort can help the administrator define a comprehensive educational program while maximizing both equipment and space.

Collaborative educational efforts should be explored. Several hospitals and a community college could develop programs in management or continuing education. The cost of the programs could be shared, and consortium efforts are regarded favorably by grantee agencies.

Premise 3: Evaluation of the educational function should include an analysis of the input, transformation, and output factors and of the feedback obtained from interacting subsystems.

The educational process should be evaluated at every phase. During the input phase, the emergence of new manpower needs to meet the demands of a changing delivery system should be monitored both inside and outside the hospital. Unmet educational needs of employees, consumers, professional students, and trustees and alternative funding mechanisms for health manpower programs also should be monitored.

During the transformation phase, particular attention should be paid to the development and evaluation of educational programs. The following questions could be useful when monitoring these activities.

1. Have the actual and perceived educational needs been assessed scientifically?

2. Do the objectives flow from the needs assessment? Are the objectives clearly stated in terms of performance so that the results of the program can be effectively evaluated?

3. Is the educational program well planned? Has a guide been developed which spells out the content, the learning experience, the various teaching methods, the teaching aids needed, and the method of evaluating the student?

4. Are the programs organized around principles of learning? Are the physical and psychological environments conducive to learning?

5. Are the faculty members well prepared and responsive to the needs of the students?

6. Are the students receiving feedback about their progress?

7. Are the programs evaluated to determine if their objectives have been attained?

8. Does the director of education keep the management staff apprised about educational program progress?

During the output phase, worker productivity, patient satisfaction, and institutional effectiveness should be evaluated. Worker productivity is high when employees understand the purpose and objective of the institution; have the skills to perform their assigned work; have an opportunity for career mobility; do not waste time or valuable resources; and have low turnover, absenteeism, accident, and grievance rates.

Patient satisfaction is high when medication errors are low; patient evaluations are positive; treatment protocol includes patient education; patient service is prompt; patient complications and infections seldom occur; and patients express confidence in the hospital personnel.

Institutional effectiveness is high when the members of the community understand the goal and objectives of the hospital; the board of trustees understands the issues involved in health care delivery; department heads think and act like managers; there are no cost overruns in manpower staffing; and the institution is responsive to collaborative ventures with other institutions in the area.

The hospital also must monitor its interaction with the delivery, education, and accreditation subsystems. The increased emphasis on preventive medicine necessitates more comprehensive consumer education programs; the development of adult learning centers facilitates independent study for hospital employees; and the stress by accrediting agencies on a quality learning environment forces the hospital educational system to continually expand and improve.

The emphasis on adult learning has fostered innovative life-long education programs such as independent and concentrated study, problem-solving projects, seminar tutorial classes, and computer-assisted instruction. In the future, hospital personnel, physicians, consumers, patients, and board members will look more and more to the hospital to share the collective knowledge it accumulates concerning the management and delivery of health services.

Hospital managers can fulfill these expectations only if they understand the hospital as an educational system and expand its educational programs designed for health manpower, consumers, and boards of trustees. Hopefully, understanding and expansion will improve patient care.

Unit III

HUMAN SKILLS FOR MANAGEMENT

A manager is a person who demonstrates positive human relations with everyone in the organization. To do this he has to understand human motivation, possess written and verbal communication skills and demonstrate effective leadership styles.

The three chapters which discuss the human skills of management address the qualities which facilitate human productivity in a work environment.

COMMUNICATION

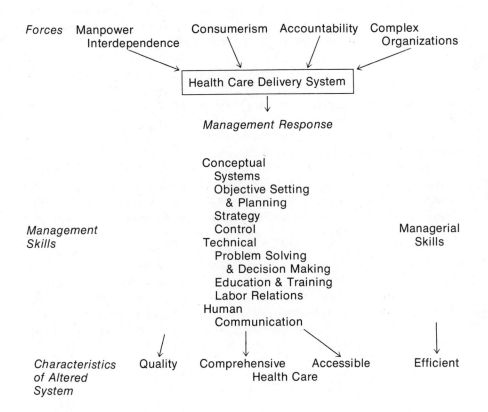

LEARNING OBJECTIVES

After carefully reading this chapter, the reader will be able to:
1. Define communication.
2. List the three types of communication.
3. List the four barriers to communication.
4. List the four factors that influence communication skill development.

167

INTRODUCTION

Complexity characterizes the health care system today. Different institutions carry out activities related to health care delivery at different levels: some removed from the patient, some rendering direct service. Examples of this are the Bureau of Health Insurance, which administers the Medicare program, and a hospital, which provides direct service to Medicare beneficiaries. Each institution has a definite function to perform, but one, the Bureau of Health Insurance, has to work through the other, the hospital, to accomplish its main goal.

This phenomenon is also true of individuals in the health care field. Some perform functions directly related to the laying-on of hands; others, such as health care managers, work through other people to accomplish the goals of patient care. As the institutions within the health care system need communication systems to carry out plans and programs, so do individuals within a health care institution need effective communication mechanisms to accomplish their work objectives.

Effective communication becomes more difficult as such external forces as accountability and consumer involvement in decision making become more pronounced. These forces influence the health-care institutions and the managers within these agencies to develop more responsive and efficient modalities for the sending and receiving of messages that result in the accomplishment of patient care. Health-care managers are finding communication skills essential as they coordinate the work of professional and nonprofessional workers with varying goals, role perceptions, and life experiences. Thus the increased complexity of the health-care environment is stimulating the manager to adapt creative ways of communicating with his employees, other managers, and the outside publics. Today more than ever, communication lies at the very heart of the management process.

THE COMMUNICATION PROCESS

Health-care managers frequently ask:

How can I get my ideas across more clearly so that patient care will be given more effectively and efficiently?

How can I reduce misunderstanding among the personnel in my department and between our department and others?

What is the best type of communication to use in a particular situation?

How can I get people to keep me informed about what is happening in my department?

What communication skills should I develop to improve the overall work performance of my department?

The answers to these questions compose an essential element of management development, since communication plays a critical role in the everyday and long-range operation of an institution. This is especially true in the case of the typical manager, who spends about 75 per cent of his time in face-to-face situations with those he supervises.

People in health care organizations communicate to provide information that will facilitate the accomplishment of work assignments and to foster understanding and rapport among employees. The middle manager is the vital element in this process. He transmits messages upward to facilitate intelligent decision-making and downward for policy implementation and organizational effectiveness. Strong environmental pressures for such goals as effective cost control and improved quality make it essential for us to use all of our skills to achieve more effective outcomes from our health services.

Communication is a process involving the sending and receiving of a message between two or more entities within a given environment. A model of the process is seen in Figure 20.

The main components of the communication process are the sender, the receiver, the message, the transfer technique, feedback and the environment. A further explanation of these elements follows.

> *Sender* — The person or group that initiates the message. The sender is a composite of past and present experiences, feeling tones, behavior patterns and social and cultural values.
> *Receiver* — the person or group that receives the message. The receiver is also a composite of past and present experiences, feeling tones, behavior patterns and social and cultural values.
> *Message* — the facts, ideas, opinions and feelings the sender conveys to the receiver.
> *Feedback* — the responses of the receiver, including all the elements of the sender's message plus modifications, substitutions, additions or even negations.
> *Transfer Technique* — the means by which the message is transmitted from the sender to the receiver. Such things as words, gestures, emotions, memorandums and letters are transfer techniques.
> *Given Environment* — the context in which the transfer of the message occurs. The environment is the internal and external surroundings of the person, group or institution.

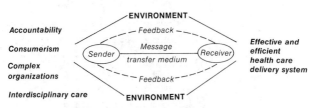

Figure 20   The communication process.

The communication process seen in this framework is changing and dynamic. When feedback occurs, the message is altered, the receiver adapts to the new message, the transfer takes on a different medium, or the environment becomes more positive or negative. Further illustrations of these ideas can be seen in the following situation.

Mrs. Wilkins, the head of the dietary department, is talking about the rising food prices with Mr. Hunt, the assistant administrator. She is attempting to tell him that the dietary department's budget will be over the projected amount for food purchases this month. Mr. Hunt responds by stressing the necessity of keeping costs down to meet a reimbursement directive established by a state agency.

Mrs. Wilkins (the sender), a registered dietitian with ten years' experience as a department head and the president of the state unit of the American Dietetic Association, *sends* this *verbal message* (food prices for staples are rising every week, which will affect the budgeted expenses for food costs) to Mr. Hunt (the receiver), a trained hospital administrator who has repeatedly stressed to all the department heads the necessity of staying within the budget. The *environment* for the message transmittal is Mr. Hunt's office on a busy Monday morning in a hospital which is operating in an external environment of a tight economy and many external constraints. Mrs. Wilkins realizes that Mr. Hunt is her immediate superior in the organization and the one who decides whether she will receive a salary increase. Mr. Hunt realizes that Mrs. Wilkins is a professional in her own right and posesses a grasp of her department's operations and has the dietary interests of the patients uppermost in her mind.

In this example, the *sender,* Mrs. Wilkins, sends a *verbal message* about a budgetary matter to the *receiver,* Mr. Hunt, within the *hospital environment.* Mr. Hunt provides *feedback,* which stresses environmental forces (rate controls) external to the individual hospital, just as Mrs. Wilkins stresses rising prices (a tight economy). Both managers seek action to meet the pressures placed upon them. At work here is not only the literal meaning of the communication but also the role and status relationships of a subordinate and superior and the professional socialization of both parties. Mrs. Wilkins could experience fear of Mr. Hunt's reaction to the news about the rising food costs and their effects on the budget. Mr. Hunt could experience frustration because the hospital's set financial plan is being altered as a result of outside forces. He knows that because of this message, adjustments will have to be made in many departments of the hospital.

Communication, then, is the process by which a sender transmits a message through a specific transfer technique to a receiver within a given environment in which feedback is encouraged.

POST TEST 9–1

Define communication.

TYPES OF COMMUNICATION

Management communication is written, oral, and nonverbal. The selection of the communication medium depends upon the message that is to be delivered.

Written Communication

In written communication, the message that is transferred between sender and receiver is an idea translated into words or symbols. Written language has constraints—it represents abstraction and semantic differentiations. In some cases, there is no shared core of experience between the sender and receiver, and as a result, the message is diluted. To overcome this problem, written communication has to project the explicit meaning of the message through the right choice of words and examples. This happens only if the writer knows his message, the purpose of the communication, and the orientation of the receiver.

In writing directives, reports and correspondence, it is essential that the communication be direct and easy to understand. The use of big words, long sentences, excessive adjectives, and involved word patterns should be kept to a minimum.

The maintenance supervisor writes and posts the following message on the boiler:

THE STEAM PRESSURE SHOULD NOT EXCEED 20 LB.

This ambiguous message will cause confusion for the maintenance workers and difficulties in monitoring this particular safety feature. A clearer way of issuing this directive is to post the following notice:

To: All Maintenance Employees
From: Mr. J. Christopher, Head of Maintenance Department
Re: Safe Steam Pressure for Boilers

In order to maintain a safe steam pressure, the boilers should not go above 20 lb. of pressure at any time. If the pressure exceeds 20 lb., stop the steam flow immediately, turn the intake valve to OFF and notify the maintenance supervisor on duty.

This written directive delineates the sender and the receiver of the message, the reason for the communication, and the specific action to be taken in the situation. In summary, written communication will be effective if the chosen words are familiar to the receiver; if ideas and recommendations are clearly stated; if the grammar, spelling, and punctuation are correct; if the receiver of the message is specified; and if the memorandum or letter is dated and signed.

Verbal Communication

Verbal communication occurs in a one-to-one situation, in small groups, or in a formal setting before an audience. This process is more interactive than is written communication, because there can be instant feedback from the sender to the receiver after the message has been delivered. A diagram of this feedback interaction is shown in Figure 21.

The sender transmits his message to the receiver through words, feelings, and attitudes—this becomes the output in the communication process. The receiver listens, assimilates the total message, and responds by giving feedback about the message to the sender. The sender may then alter the message because of this additional information.

In a verbal setting, the sender and receiver bring directly to the communication situation their own feelings, values, and expectations; thus interaction occurs only when a common core of experience is established between the listener and the receiver.

> The director of nursing service, in talking to a group of nurse-aide trainees, explains that they may feel insecure on the patient floors until they become accustomed to the hospital. She tells them that she experienced this apprehension when she was a young student nurse. This remark puts the trainees at ease and helps them to realize that other people have had the same feelings as they. They begin to drop the defenses caused by their anxiety and listen to the remarks of the nursing director.

In verbal communication, the transfer medium is the spoken word. Since words have different meanings for different people, they should be selected specifically for each particular communication setting. A nurse giving directions for insulin injection to an elderly diabetic patient does not use complicated technical terms to describe the procedure. Instead, she selects the terms familiar to the patient, taking into consideration his cultural and social orientation.

Congruence is also essential for clear verbal communication. Since the whole person communicates, a person's attitudes and feelings manifest themselves in the process. In other words, it is difficult to deliver a happy message in a convincing manner when one is angry or hostile. Finally, verbal communication is effective only when feedback is obtained continually. This assures that the message delivered is being received accurately.

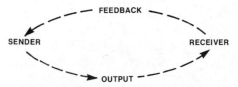

Figure 21   Verbal communication interaction.

Nonverbal Communication

Body language, or nonverbal communication, is an important aspect of the communication process. Such things as the manner of speech, gestures, facial expressions, and bodily postures are clues about the way the communication is progressing. A glance at one's wrist watch during an interview, impatient tapping of fingers on a desk, frowning, and yawning tell more about the true viewpoint of the sender or the receiver than do the words that are being said.

POST-TEST 9–2

List the three types of communication.

COMMUNICATION BARRIERS

Barriers in the communication process can be physical, cultural, psychological, or organizational. These barriers interfere and, at times, stop the communication process. This process is shown in Figure 22.

Physical Barriers

Some of the physical communication barriers are environmental stimuli, room arrangements, and, in the case of written communication, the presentation of the written message.

Unnecessary noise in the area in which communication is occurring can block the sending and receiving of messages. When a physician holds a conversation with a patient in an area adjoining construction activity, energy is drained from both participants, and weakened communication results. To counteract the noise barrier, quiet surroundings should be selected for communication whenever possible.

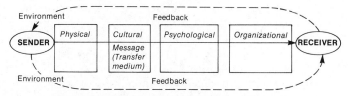

Figure 22 Barriers to the communication process.

Temperature extremes can also detract from the communication interaction. When a person is too hot or cold, he is distracted from the immediate task of listening or talking.

The physical arrangements of a room impede or facilitate communication. The presence of a large desk between the sender and the receiver acts as a barrier in some communication situations. In a department head–employee conversation, the desk can be seen by the employee as a symbol of authority and status and may influence the manner in which he responds to the messages being transmitted. In group discussions, arranging chairs in a classroom style hinders the exchange of ideas. Likewise, placing chairs in a conversational style facilitates discussion.

In written communication, poor typing, unattractive paper, misspelled words, and improper grammar detract from the message that is being conveyed. The written message represents the sender to the person or group receiving the communication. Therefore, it should be attractive and presentable.

Cultural Barriers

Cultural barriers are those impediments to communication that spring from the socioeconomic class, mores, language, and roles people bring to the work situation.

The socioeconomic class of a person determines the way in which he perceives the world and makes value judgments. Within the health care setting, people with varying socioeconomic backgrounds come together, especially people who have strong ethnic and religious practices. An illustration of this follows.

> Jim Goldstein has been employed as a physical therapy assistant. Mr. Crowns, the department head, schedules Jim to work every Saturday. Since this is a day of quiet and rest for orthodox Jewish people, the assignment creates anxiety for the new employee, who reacts with sullenness when he sees the time sheet. The department head is confused by this reaction.

In this example, the religious beliefs of an employee interfered with the assignment of a task. Sensitivity to these situations can alleviate many tense situations for employees and keep communication channels open.

The use of language is also conditioned by the cultural background of people. We learn the meaning of words by relating them to our experiences. The phrase "emergency room" may mean something entirely different to a nurse and to a parent whose child swallowed a safety pin and was rushed to the hospital. The simplest words have an infinite number of meanings for both the sender and the receiver and should be thoughtfully chosen in order to be understood by both.

One problem frequently occurring in semantics is the use of stereotypes and labels. Such labels falsely associate objects, people, and events that are not identical. Because of cultural conditioning, some people have fixed reactions to certain groups. For example, the chief physical therapist feels that all young people are lazy and irresponsible. The laundry director believes that labor unions are disruptive. Often because of stereotyping, we fail to differentiate between particular individuals or events and distort our judgment and communication.

In dealing with questions of semantics, it is important to get feedback continually. If what you are saying is being decoded and assimilated erroneously, communication will not occur. Such phrases as "Is this what you mean...?" or "If I understand what you are saying..." are helpful in minimizing the chances of drawing the wrong conclusions.

Role conflicts and role ambiguities can also cause communication problems. Individuals within an organization occupy certain positions, and their performance is determined by the expectations, social norms, and rules of the organization. Besides having a particular role within the work situation, a person can also play other roles. For example, the business office manager can be a supervisor, father, husband, member of the chamber of commerce, and P.T.A. president. All of these roles demand different behaviors and can impinge on one another. If there is a sick child in the family, the paternal role may interfere with and dominate the supervisory role while the man is at work.

Role conflict within the work situation also becomes evident when a supervisor exerts pressure on an employee for performance based on his expectations of the particular job. This is illustrated in the following incident.

> The chief medical technologist of a 400-bed hospital becomes upset when the hematology technologist who has just been hired does not perform a certain number of analyses each hour. This volume of work production is necessary to meet the service demands on the laboratory. The hematology technologist feels a great deal of pressure for this type of work performance because he is used to a slower pace and lighter work output; his last job assignment was in a 50-bed hospital.

In the example, the chief technologist had one expectation of the hematology technologist's performance and the technologist had another. Role conflicts, then, can arise from the necessity for people to play more than one role and from dissonant expectations about role performance. Communication is affected because of the tension and anxiety produced by the conflict. To eliminate this barrier, role expectations for employees should be clarified when they are first employed. When conflict is evident, the causes of the tense situation should be discussed with the supervisor and the employee.

Psychological Barriers

Psychological barriers manifest themselves through a narrow self-concept, negative feelings, and personality clashes.

A person's self-concept can at times act as a communication barrier. Often the view a person has of himself is not the same as the one he presents to others. The person's real self and self-concept may be incongruent because people are not always aware of all of the emotional, social, psychological, and cultural attributes of their personalities, even though these influence the way they view the world and the manner in which they communicate with others.

> The director of housekeeping perceives one of the unit maids as a person with organizational and leadership skills and recommends her for a supervisory position. The unit maid sees herself as insecure, afraid of making any mistakes, and shy around strangers. When told she has been recommended for a supervisory position, she immediately becomes anxious and frightened and makes excuses as to why she should not have the promotion.

Negative feelings are another communication barrier. Listening is impaired when we feel defensive. We listen for implication rather than for the message the sender is delivering. Hostility in particular can inhibit the communication process, since the hostile person is trying to strike out at the other during the exchange.

Personality clashes can impede the sending and receiving of messages. Issues can be personified rather than handled in terms of organizational needs. When there are power struggles to gain control of a group or situation, the communication process can break down completely.

Organizational Barriers

Communication problems are evident when organizations increase in size. In a small hospital with only 50 employees, the administrator can send a message to his workers with very little effort. He knows them personally, and if he wishes to communicate with them, he has only to walk through the hospital and do so. In a large organization, however, such face-to-face transmission of messages is not feasible, and less personal methods must be used. Total communication effectiveness suffers in larger organizations because the impersonal methods of communication do not afford the same opportunities for feedback that face-to-face communication does.

Another problem caused by an increase in the number of employees lies in the nature of the formal communication system required in a larger organization. Message distortion is increased when messages are transmitted through a number of people. Large organizations also create barriers of distance between departments and people, which inhibit the free exchange of ideas.

In summary, barriers in the communication process can be physical, cultural, psychological, or organizational. These barriers interfere with and at times can stop communication entirely.

POST-TEST 9–3

List the four barriers to communication.

COMMUNICATION SKILL DEVELOPMENT

Successful communication depends upon a reinforcing environment, the development of sending and receiving skills, appropriate message and channel choices, and a well-defined feedback mechanism.

Communication is enhanced when the individuals in the work'situation are treated with respect and dignity. It flourishes when they are praised and recognized for their accomplishments and are not made to feel that they are constantly being evaluated. A positive climate gives employees an opportunity to develop and not be afraid of open communication. The environment improves when supervisors are available to talk to employees and listen to their complaints. Subordinates should also be encouraged to participate in the solution of group problems when they suggest something worthwhile.

People who listen well encourage people to talk freely, obtain information about the causes of problems, and reinforce others' self-worth. The head nurse who is available to listen to the nurses on her floor usually has a ward of satisfied patients, low turnover, and high employee morale. In developing listening skills, one should show a genuine interest in the person to whom one is listening, pay attention to what is being said, and express empathy with the other person's viewpoint. It is well to be silent when there is a need to do so and not worry that there are lapses, or quiet periods, in the conversation.

In order to assure the correct message, channel choices, and appropriate feedback, formal communication channels should be present within the health care organization. Horizontal communication is enhanced by realistic organizational charts, job descriptions, and joint interdepartmental meetings and projects.

Upward communication occurs when clear communication channels are delineated and through the use of opinion polls. Downward communication flourishes when the communication practices of each department are evaluated, when group planning sessions are held, and when the employees are given an opportunity to voice their opinions.

Today's health care system is composed of many institutions functioning at different levels to provide health services. Institutional complexity is coupled with social, political, and economic forces that affect health care facilities.

The health care manager functioning in this complicated milieu finds it necessary to develop technical, conceptual, and human skills to carry out his management function. Communication is one of the most important of these. Through the sending and receiving of written, verbal, and nonverbal messages, the middle manager accomplishes work related to patient-care programs and stabilizes employee relations.

A manager knowledgeable about the communication process guards against the physical, cultural, psychological, and organizational barriers that negate effective interaction within the work environment. He builds strong communication systems that insure a positive environment and vertical and horizontal message channels.

The development of effective communication skills for health care managers assures a delivery system that is responsive to the clients within the health care institution and to the society at large that is demanding accountability.

POST-TEST 9–4

List the four factors that influence communication skill development.

SUMMARY

Communication is a process involving the sending and receiving of a message between two or more entities within a given environment. Management communication is written, oral, and nonverbal and can be impeded by several barriers. Finally, communication skill is developed through a reinforcing environment and adequate feedback.

RECAP EXERCISE 9

Springhill Hospital is a 500-bed hospital located in a large urban section of Pennsylvania. The population in the surrounding area consists of poor blacks and Puerto Ricans. Although the hospital has been in the area for 50 years, it has never had an organized community relations program. One week ago, four representatives from the Keystone Rangers group contacted the hospital administrator about having a well-baby clinic set up in the hospital to provide routine physical examinations to infants, conduct educational sessions for new mothers, and give nutritional counseling to families with small children.

The administrator received the approval of the board for the establishment of the clinic. He asked the director of nursing service, the dietary department supervisor, and the outpatient department supervisor to plan for the clinic with the community groups and the departments in the hospital.

1. What forces outside the hospital influenced the decision to develop a well-baby clinic?
2. In the transaction between the hospital administrator and the representative of the Keystone Rangers,
   a. What was the message?
   b. Who was the sender? the receiver?
   c. What type of communication was used?
   d. What barriers could have been present?
3. In order to develop the well-baby clinic, what communication systems will have to be developed?
   a. Within the hospital?
   b. Outside the hospital?
   c. Within the clinic?
4. What communication skills will have to be developed by the health care managers who will be involved either directly or indirectly with the clinic?

REFERENCES

1. Bassett, Glen A.: *Communication Both Ways.* New York, American Management Association, 1967.
2. Burby, Raymond, J.: *Communicating with People: The Supervisor's Introduction to Verbal Communication and Decision Making.* Reading, Mass., Addison-Wesley Publishing Co., 1970.
3. Cohen, A. M.: Changing small-group communication networks. *Administrative Science Quarterly 6*:443–462, 1962.
4. Davis, Keith: *Human Relations at Work: The Dynamics of Organizational Behavior,* 3rd ed. New York, McGraw-Hill Book Co., 1967.
5. Emergy, J. C.: *Organizational Planning and Control Systems.* New York, Macmillan Inc., 1969.
6. Guetzkow, H.: Communication in organizations. In March, J. G. (ed.): *Handbook of Organizations.* Chicago, Rand-McNally, 1965, pp. 534–573.
7. Hainmann, T., and Scott, W. G.: *Management in the Modern Organization.* Boston, Houghton Mifflin, 1970.
8. Laird, Dugan: *Business Writing Skills: A Workbook.* Reading, Mass., Addison-Wesley Publishing Co., 1970.
9. Reed, James M., and Silleck, Anne: *Better Business Letters—A Programmed Book to Develop Skill in Writing.* Reading, Mass., Addison-Wesley Publishing Co., 1969.
10. Rogers, C. R., and Roethlisberger, F. J.: Barriers and gateways to communication. *Harvard Business Review 30*:46–52, 1952.
11. Thayer, L.: *Communication and Communication Systems.* Homewood, Ill., Richard D. Irwin, Inc., 1968.
12. Vardaman, George: *Effective Communication of Ideas.* New York, McGraw-Hill Book Co., 1967.

MOTIVATION

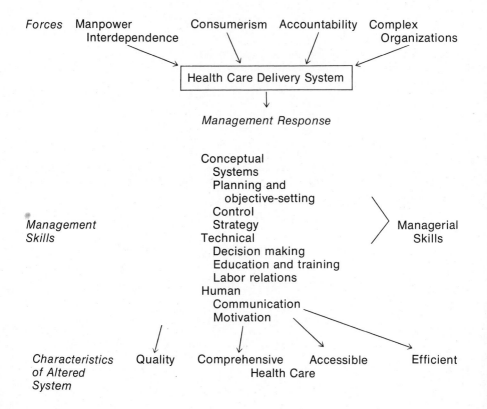

LEARNING OBJECTIVES

After reading this chapter, the reader will be able to:
1. Define motivation.
2. Describe four factors present in the motivational process.
3. List four behavioral manifestations of frustration.
4. Define achievement motivation.
5. List three ways of building achievement motivation in your organization.

INTRODUCTION

Human behavior stems from factors meaningful to the individual in his environment. Most behavior can be traced to people's attitudes and desires to satisfy basic needs and attain individual goals. Psychologists emphasize different aspects of individual behavior, but all stress the complexity of human motivation—that energetic source which steers behavior to the attainment of purposive activity. Constant interaction occurs between attitudes, goal definition, and satisfaction. Frustration results when goal achievement is blocked. When dealing with a frustrated worker, a manager can facilitate positive motivation and eliminate goal frustration; thus he creates an environment that effectively satisfies employees' needs while getting the work done.

MOTIVATIONAL PROCESS

Motivation is the process governing choices among alternative forms of activity. The motivational process is influenced by a person's attitudes and needs. These forces produce the definition and accomplishment of a goal and are manifested through selected activities. A diagram of the entire process is illustrated in Figure 23.

The motivational process, then, comprises the interactions whereby a person with a specific set of attitudes defines needs, goals, and goal accomplishment through the choice of specified activities.

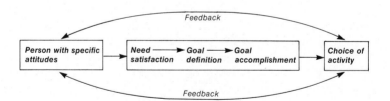

Figure 23 The motivational process.

POST-TEST 10–1

Define motivation.

Attitudes

An attitude may be defined as an inclination to act based on the individual's interpretation of a situation, person, or idea. Attitudes constitute an individual's likes and dislikes. Attitudes possess overtones that may vary from positive to neutral to negative in intensity.

Faced with a change of routine, an employee may feel, "Well, I suppose it won't hurt to try it the new way," or, "I refuse to change this procedure one more time. Old Man Higgins is going to have to make up his mind." In the first instance, the person does not feel strongly one way or the other about the change, whereas in the second example, the employee's attitude about the change and his boss is negative.

Several factors influence attitude formation. The most important are a person's biological make-up, the significant people in his environment, and the groups with which he associates.

In terms of biological factors, sex, age, height, race, weight, and body type are important determinants of attitudes that contribute to overall personality structure.

The significant people in a person's environment who help to shape his attitudes are the immediate family and relatives. For instance, a person may become a Democrat because of his father, or he may value hard work because its importance was stressed in his home during childhood. If he receives love and reinforcement in the home environment, he will probably perceive himself as a person of worth. But if he is constantly downgraded by his parents, spouse, or children, he will consider himself inferior.

The social and economic class into which a person is born affects his attitudes and establishes patterns for future interpersonal relationships. The upper class takes for granted refinement of living and preferential treatment, whereas in middle and lower class families, the children are expected to work hard in order to succeed.

Besides the family and its value system, an individual's attitudes stem partly from the groups with which he affiliates. For the child, there is the play group; later on, there will be his school friends, his Sunday school group, and, when he reaches maturity, his work group. The work group, the hospital department, and the total institution influence a person's attitudes about work, human values, and his own self-image. Often, the main influence on a person's attitudes is not the entire group, but dominant people within it, such as a friend or neighbor.

From a management viewpoint, an understanding of individual attitudes becomes a critical factor in motivating employees. No matter what factors caused their development, attitudes become deep-seated attributes of the individual's character because they are learned and acquired over a long period of time. If an employee's attitudes lead to desirable, constructive, cooperative behavior, the manager will want to strengthen and encourage them. However, if they result in undesirable behavior, the supervisor's problem is that of trying to change the attitudes or modify the employee's environment so that his behavior changes. In short, attitudes help determine the individual route that the person takes for the satisfaction of his needs.

Need Satisfaction

Another component of the motivation process is the individual's desire to satisfy needs and life goals. The goals of a person stem from his unfulfilled needs. Hence, hunger will lead to a major goal—eating. As hunger decreases, another need emerges with an attendant goal definition. There are various categories of needs, some of which the majority of people share and others that just a few people completely realize.

The categories that most humans share in common are the satisfaction of sensory and safety needs. The most basic and most powerful human needs are for oxygen, food, liquid, shelter, sex, and sleep. A person who is lacking food, self-esteem, and love will usually demand food first and, until his need is satisfied, will ignore or push all other desires into the background.

Once the physiological needs are sufficiently satisfied, the safety needs emerge: the need for predictability of environment and protection from physical harm, a continuing income and employment, and some form of stable routine. These needs are met through adequate housing, a dependable job, and habitual activities of daily living.

When the sensory and safety requirements are met, desires for love and a feeling of belonging emerge. A person wants affectionate relationships with others; he wants a place in the group and acceptance by others. A person deprived of emotional satisfaction over an extended period of time can become incapable of relating in a positive manner with others.

If a person is well-grounded in love, he begins to seek competence and mastery of a particular area. He also strives for independence and freedom. A person with adequate self-esteem gains confidence and may become more productive; a person without it suffers from feelings of inferiority. Finally, a person who has satisfied his sensory and emotional needs reaches out for self-actualization. This is the desire to become what one is capable of becoming. One who is fully integrated seeks to realize his potential to the fullest.

The need satisfaction and attainment process follows an organization unique to each individual. At any point one need becomes more powerful and more prominent than others in influencing the individual's behavior. As one need satisfaction occurs, others replace it. As long as the original need gets enough gratification, it remains quiet and is much less likely to rouse the individual to action than is one of the still unsatisfied needs.

POST-TEST 10–2

1. Define four factors present in the motivational process.
2. Mary Peters grew up in a middle-class family that valued hard work and saving money. She has just finished college and wants to get a permanent job so she can begin to save some money and establish her own household. She comes to the hospital to apply for the position of assistant office manager.

Isolate the factors in the motivational process that prompted Mary Peters to apply for the job of assistant office manager.

Factors	Explanation
Personality	
Specific attitudes	
Needs	
Goal	
Accomplishment of goal	
Choice of activity	

FRUSTRATION AND ITS MANIFESTATION

When an individual accomplishes his goals, his needs are satisfied and his positive attitudes reinforced. On the other hand, if his chosen course of action hampers goal fulfillment, conflict and frustration result.

The behavior patterns most frequently associated with frustration on the job are alternative action, withdrawal, striking back, and passivity.

Alternative Action

The most positive response to frustration is some type of action that substitutes one positive goal for another to satisfy a need. If the person can look at the conflict objectively and decide on a positive course of action, little harm occurs. For example, a dietitian realizes that she cannot run for office in her professional organization because she lacks public-speaking ability, so she may enroll in a public-speaking class at the university. A licensed practical nurse finds herself unable to work in the emergency room because the high stress situations upset her, so she becomes skilled in the care of medical patients.

Employees who handle frustration positively take the initiative in discussing their particular conflict and ask for suggestions on resolving problems. Although the handling of frustration in a positive way is preferred, such negative behavior as withdrawal, striking out, and passivity also occurs.

Withdrawal

Often a person will not come to grips with a conflicting situation but runs away from it. For instance, one of the medical record employees has ideas for improving the abstracting of the Professional Activity Survey form. Every time she comes up with a new procedure her supervisor tells her, "You're not paid to reorganize the department. Just do the abstracting as you have been shown." The person responds by taking frequent sick days and finally quits.

Daydreaming also produces escape. Within limits, it may be acceptable behavior; however, when it becomes a substitute for reality, it detracts from effectiveness. A maid in the housekeeping department who has been told repeatedly by her supervisor that her floor-cleaning procedures fail to meet the standards of the department fantasizes being promoted to the chief housekeeper position by the hospital administrator.

The person with withdrawal patterns often is late for work and frequently absent. At times, he seems unable to concentrate and lets his mind wander. Often he changes jobs to escape unpleasant situations arising from the work situation.

Finally, a person can withdraw by reverting to childlike behavior and feelings. Often, he regresses to a former state that was happier than the present one. For example, the new assistant director of the pharmacy may spend most of his time filling prescriptions rather than trying to learn his management duties of evaluating employees, working on the budget, and attending committee meetings.

Striking Out

Anger or antagonism toward the barrier that prevents the accomplishment of a goal constitutes another negative way of expressing frustration. This anger may be shown either directly against the person or object blocking the goal or indirectly against some other person, the frustrated person himself, or an unrelated object. If a laundry worker feels that her immediate supervisor blocked her chances for getting a raise, she may pick arguments with the supervisor, start rumors about him, and in general, make him look bad. Another employee in the same area who didn't get a raise may continue to be pleasant toward his supervisor but go home and be angry with his wife and children. Aggressive behavior further manifests itself in complaints, grievances, damage to equipment, and friction between employees. Aggression offers a temporary relief to frustration of goal satisfaction but often results in tension and negative human relationships.

Passivity

Listlessness, lack of interest, and apathy are common manifestations of a passive reaction to frustration. Mr. Stokes, the night security man, missed several opportunities to be promoted. When he discusses this situation, he either says, "I don't care" or tells people that he was not promoted "because one of the other security men made him look bad." Employees showing passive behavior blame the equipment, the working hours, or the supervisor for their mistakes and failures.

The passive individual becomes pessimistic about his future. He continually finds excuses for his failures and no longer tries to improve, gain new experiences, or grow as a person. This is shown in the following example.

> Ted Johnson, an orderly in the emergency room of Memorial Hospital, well-liked by his fellow employees, has recently been elected an officer of the Employees' Credit Union. He and two of his friends are planning a trip to Yellowstone Park for the summer. Three days ago, Ted learned that his house needs a new furnace, which will cost around $500. He will have to use his vacation money to pay for it. Still upset about the news, he goes to the bowling alley to play in the hospital tournament. The Memorial Hospital team is playing in the semifinals. Ted can't get started and throws 7–10 splits all evening.

In this case, Ted's vacation plans have been blocked by the need for a new furnace. He is frustrated and shows it in his behavior.

POST-TEST 10–3

List four ways in which frustration can be revealed in your behavior.

PRODUCING ACHIEVEMENT MOTIVATION

Achievement motivation is the desire to accomplish positive goals. This desire grows in an environment that provides the opportunity for personal responsibility, gives feedback about job performance, and rewards a job well done.

Achievement motivation can be enhanced in the work environment if the manager understands different views about humanity, the determinants of job satisfaction, and the methods of dealing with frustration.

The Nature of Humans

Philosophies of motivation depend on one's viewpoint about the nature of people and their behavior in the workplace. Two points of view prevail: the concept of the authority-dominated and of the self-actualizing environment to produce motivation.

AUTHORITY-DOMINATED ENVIRONMENT

This philosophy of motivation views people as being opposed to work and lacking the capacity for self-direction and personal responsibility. It states that workers would rather be told what to do than think for themselves.

This pessimistic view of people has its genesis in the notion that a person is basically rebellious and uncooperative and should be strictly controlled. Managers who subscribe to this idea hold that the employee has a fixed nature, is prone to inefficiency, and will waste time unless he is properly programmed. They also believe that the employee's main motivation is economic, with money being the one incentive that will induce him to work. As a result, the employee is seen as lazy, needing tight controls and external supervision to make him overcome his natural desire to avoid work. In accommodating to this view of man, the organizational environment is characterized by specialization of personnel, impersonality, a hierarchy of authority relationships, entry and advancement by competitive examination, written policies, and the strict adherence to rules and procedures.

The manager who believes that people should be in a controlled environment and that they are motivated principally by economic incentives does little to assist the employee in self-development. Instead, emphasis is placed on work output and monetary rewards for performance, and authoritarian relationships are the modus operandi for the institution.

SELF-ACTUALIZING ENVIRONMENT

The second philosophy stresses that a person is a creative social being with worth and goodness, who gains satisfaction from working and cooperating with other people. Management should provide people with the opportunity to grow and mature into human beings who can realize their own goals best by working for the success of the organization. In this situation, there is an interdependence of managers and employees—they are united in the accomplishment of the goals of the organization and the individual goals of the people in it.

Determinants of Job Satisfaction

The determinants of job satisfaction in the work situation are related to supervision, influence in the decision making, the work group, job content, and wages.

SUPERVISION

An employee's relationship with his immediate supervisor influences his morale, general satisfaction, and productivity on the job.

A supervisor who is interested in his employees acts as a facilitator for the attainment of rewards and the avoidance of punishment. The most satisfied workers are trained to perform their jobs well with supervisors who recognize their accomplishments. When the supervisor subscribes to participative management, he becomes primarily a consultant rather than a rule enforcer, and the employee then receives more challenge to heighten his work interest.

On the other hand, poor supervision causes employee dissatisfaction, turnover, accidents, and low morale.

INFLUENCE IN DECISION-MAKING

Employee satisfaction is positively associated with the degree to which employees are permitted an opportunity to participate in decision making.

The basic managerial and motivational problem in organizations today is our failure to encourage decision making and responsibility commitment. The typical organization encourages people to take problems to supervisors and higher-level managers for solution. More effective organizations encourage employees to bring solutions for ratification and implementation.

The supervisor who encourages participation does so by asking for advice and help on problems relating to the work; he gives orders in the form of questions, where possible, and refrains from excessive interference and oversupervision. He delegates tasks that could be done better at a lower level. Concomitantly, the supervisor encourages decision making in his subordinates and shares communication about problems and activities in the institution and the progress of the various projects that are operative in the department or work unit. Creative decision-making by employees should be rewarded by promotion and recognition to further reinforce this behavior within the work group.

THE WORK GROUP

People, as social beings, need to be in contact with their fellow human beings. In the work situation, face-to-face contact does influence worker productivity and satisfaction. If the employees perceive their work group as assisting them in receiving rewards, they will have positive reactions about it; on the other hand, if the work group is seen as destructive, negative reaction toward the group follows. Workers also require interaction with each other on the job.

Another important variable is the acceptance of the employee by the other members of the group. The manner in which a new employee relates with his fellow workers may determine to a large degree his satisfaction with his job, his attitude toward his employer and the hospital, productivity, the quality of work, and even the length of time he remains with the institution.

Groups attract people through their goals and programs and their position in the community. A hospital serves a necessary function in the community by providing a humane service to the sick and injured. People working in a hospital are usually viewed by other citizens as performing a needed service. Therefore, working for a hospital brings prestige to its employees.

JOB CONTENT

Besides the reinforcement of the supervisor and the satisfying relationships within the work group, the content of the job influences the motivation of the employees. The number and character of the functions that individual workers are called upon to perform vary tremendously from one work role to another. For example, the duties of the doctor, the assembly-line worker, the policeman, and the corporation president differ extensively in knowledge needed and skill specification.

A distinction must also be made between job content and job context. Job context refers to the environment of the work scene and deals with security, wages, supervision, social aspects of the job, and working conditions; job content deals with the work itself, achievement, and advancement possibilities. In analyzing the content of the job, it should be kept in mind that repetitive tasks cause dissatisfaction in the workers. Boredom is less likely to arise when the form of activity changes at suitable times within the period of work. For example, the people assigned to wash dishes in the dietary department who have other duties to perform, such as setting up trays for meals, become less dissatisfied with their jobs than those who are assigned to the dishwasher all day. Boredom is further reduced when suitable rest pauses (such as the coffee and lunch breaks) are introduced, giving both needed physical activity changes and opportunities to socialize with fellow employees.

When feasible, the employee should have some control over the work methods. Workers frequently discover methods of work better suited to their requirements than the ones prescribed. If they have the freedom to experiment with work methods, new and more satisfying ways of performing work assignments may develop. Again, the expectation that the worker can offer solutions and not problems applies.

Workers should also have some control over the pace of their work. The pace at which a worker performs his job may be regulated either socially or mechanically. The term "close supervision" is typically used to refer to a relationship between supervisor and worker in which the presence of the supervisor closely constrains the worker's choice of work pace. Presumably, workers subject to close supervision have less freedom to vary their work pace without incurring penalties than those subject to more general supervision. Controlled conveyor systems also regulate the speed with which the worker carries out his job.

Many studies show that workers derive satisfaction from jobs that permit them to use their skills and abilities. Finally, the worker wants to succeed in his job; he wants to believe that a task requires abilities that he values and believes himself to possess.

WAGES

Persistent controversy revolves around the importance of wages to workers. Many managers stress the importance of the size of the pay check in determining a worker's job satisfaction and the probability of his remaining in his job.

Satisfaction stemming from wages depends not only on the absolute amount of the money received but also on the relationship between that amount and some standard of comparison used by the individual. For example, Sam and John began work at the same time as orderlies in the central supply department. Sam discovers that John receives a higher salary than he. Sam may protest this inequity to the personnel director or engage in other types of less productive behavior.

Monetary incentives may be effective in increasing productivity in many organizations today, although some types of work (professional, artistic) seem less suited for this type of reward. Professionals obtain great satisfaction by bettering their own performance. Since professionals enjoy higher levels of income than other workers, their income needs may be less pressing.

Dealing with Frustration on the Job

The work situation contains many sources of frustration. Therefore, the manager should be alert to possibilities for preventing or reducing work conflict and tension. However, when conditions prevail that inevitably cause frustration, the supervisor should work to relieve them.

When employees find their jobs satisfying in terms of personal and work goals, frustration occurs less frequently. Employees tend to experience frustration when they do not feel that their efforts are appreciated and approved by their supervisor. Periodic performance reviews with the employee reduce frustration from this source. For the manager, periodic performance reviews provide opportunities to get to know his employees better and to learn more about their attitudes, motivation, and conflicts.

Jobs can be made more satisfying if the employees feel that they can participate in the decision-making process within the organization. Group discussions with the employees facilitate this effort, reveal frustrations quickly, and help to relieve tension. The employees find out what is going on and why; they get a better idea of what to expect in their work and have a chance to ask questions and to make suggestions. Group discussion creates a freer atmosphere. Furthermore, the information that the supervisor gains from a discussion helps him to become familiar with the group's problems in general and with some of the specific problems of individual employees.

Frustration can be further relieved on the job by helping the employees to establish realistic goals and by changing frustrating situations.

Often goal change offers the only way that a person can overcome his frustration. Frustrated people generally need help, but they either don't know it or avoid facing the fact. Therefore, direct advice might be resisted. Consequently, one should first discuss the problem with the person, and let him talk about it freely, so as to understand the situation from his point of view. In the early stages of discussion, he may not even be able to see his problem clearly. Prudent counseling can help the individual to gain insight and reach a point where behavior evaluation is not threatening. When the person seems to be receptive to the matters under discussion, a more appropriate and attainable goal may be evident or suggested.

Often a frustrating situation on a job can be altered to make the work environment more pleasant for the employees. In some instances, this may be done by reducing the work load, or giving the individual assignments that he handles more ably. In other instances, he may need additional help. The supervisor should provide the employee with information concerning opportunities in the company. A fair system of evaluating the ability and potential of employees can be used to provide them with the kind of work they are best suited for, as well as opportunities for promotion.

POST-TEST 10–4

1. Define achievement motivation.
2. List three ways of building achievement motivation in your organization.

SUMMARY

The effective manager is one who recognizes that every individual's behavior is unique because of his particular attitudes, needs, and goals. Each individual is motivated by the need for the satisfaction of particular desires at a particular time. Because motivation is inherent in people, the task of the manager is to unleash and harness the existing energy. This is accomplished by helping another to examine his own point of view and how he arrived at it. The manager can effect positive motivation by recognizing frustration and trying to eliminate it, while reinforcing achievement behavior.

RECAP EXERCISE 10

Jack Andrews is a good department head. Now, with his promotion and transfer to the administrative staff, Mr. Goldstein, the chief executive officer, hires Mary Haney as the new director of the x-ray department.

Ms. Haney will start on the job next week. Four of the x-ray department employees are discussing their new supervisor and what they hope shee will be like.

Nancy:	Wonder what Ms. Haney is going to be like.
John:	I hope she believes in giving raises. I sure could use one now.
Sally:	I'd almost forego a raise in order not to lose some say in how this department is run. Jack was so good about discussing problems and plans with us.
Peter:	If this Ms. Haney upsets our work groups, I may quit. I like the team I'm with now, and I don't want to be moved.
Sally:	Me too! I sure hope she lets me stick to the job I'm doing now. I've just devised some faster ways to process the film, and I want to keep working on the darkroom procedures.
John:	Yeah, and I hope she'll tell us when we're doing all right and doesn't always put the blame on us when anything goes wrong.
Peter:	One thing I'm going to ask for is that she have the department painted. This place looks dreadful!
Nancy:	I hope she's like Jack and lets us off for those continuing education classes. I've been getting a lot out of them, and I bet the technologists who go to all of them will receive advancement in the association.
Peter:	I feel the same way about it. If the boss appreciates you and sees that you're trying to do a good job, she should let you know about it. And if she doesn't like what you do, she should tell you why and help you do better. That's the only way you can learn.
Nancy:	And she ought to take time to explain things. I like to know what's going on and what's expected of me.
Sally:	Well, we'll know the story Monday.

1. List some of the things the employees in the x-ray department wanted. Put these answers in the column marked "what." After you have defined the determinants of job satisfaction for these employees, fill in the reasons why they want these things.

	What	Why
Example	Good working conditions	Recognition

2. What types of strategy should Ms. Haney use in motivating the employees in the x-ray department?

REFERENCES

1. Blake, R. R., and Mouton, J. S.: *Building a Dynamic Corporation through Grid Organization Development*. Reading, Mass., Addison-Wesley Publishing Co., 1969.
2. Contemporary Publishing: *Motivating Personnel and Managing Conflict*. New York, Contemporary Publishing Co., 1974.
3. Cyert, Richard, and March, James G.: *A Behavioral Theory of the Firm*. Englewood Cliffs, N. J., Prentice-Hall, Inc., 1963.
4. Gardner, John W.: *Self-Renewal: The Individual and the Innovative Society*. New York, Harper and Row, 1964.
5. Gillermann, S.: *Motivation and Productivity*. New York, American Management Association, 1963.
6. Golembrewski, Robert T.: *Men, Management and Morality: Toward a New Organizational Ethic*. New York, McGraw-Hill Book Co., 1965.
7. Hackman, Ray C.: *The Motivated Working Adult*. New York, American Management Association, 1969.
8. Herzberg, F.: One more time: How do you motivate employees? *Harvard Business Review* 46:53, 1968.
9. Kiesler, Charles A.: *Attitude Change*. New York, John Wiley & Sons, Inc., 1969.
10. Likert, Renesis: *New Patterns of Management*. New York, McGraw-Hill Book Co., 1961.
11. Maslow, A. H.: *Motivation and Personality*. New York, Harper and Row, 1954.
12. McCoy, James T.: *Beyond Motivation*. New York, Jeffrey Norton Publishers, 1973.
13. McGregor, Douglas: *The Human Side of Enterprise*. New York, McGraw Hill Book Co., 1958.
14. Vroom, V. H.: *Work and Motivation*. New York, John Wiley & Sons, Inc., 1964.
15. Wasmuth, William J.: *Human Resources Administration*. Boston, Houghton Mifflin Co., 1970.

INTERPERSONAL RELATIONSHIPS

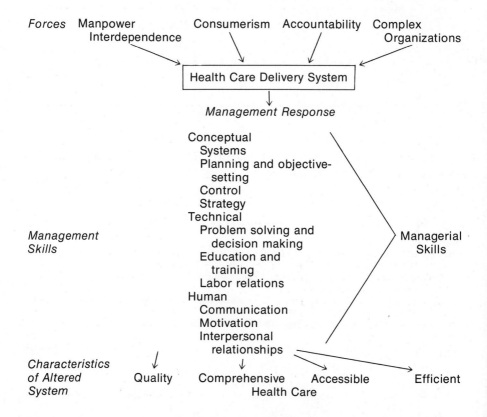

Forces Manpower Consumerism Accountability Complex
       Interdependence   Organizations

Health Care Delivery System

Management Response

Conceptual
  Systems
  Planning and objective-
    setting
  Control
  Strategy
Technical
  Problem solving and
    decision making
  Education and
    training
  Labor relations
Human
  Communication
  Motivation
  Interpersonal
    relationships

Management Skills

Managerial Skills

Characteristics of Altered System Quality Comprehensive Accessible Efficient
                               Health Care

LEARNING OBJECTIVES

After carefully reading this chapter, the reader will be able to:
1. List the four personal qualifications for leadership.
2. List the three types of leadership styles.
3. List the four factors that make each employee a unique individual.
4. Define the two kinds of work groups.
5. Discuss why the group is important for the individual.
6. List four ways in which the manager can facilitate group effort.
7. List three ways that a manager can show positive regard for other people.
8. Discuss two ways that a manager can facilitate a climate for development for his employees.

INTRODUCTION

Both harmonious and conflictive relations among individuals and groups provide the basis for individual and institutional effectiveness. Harmonious interaction among people in an organization makes it function, and positive human relationships can make a pleasant and productive environment. Conflictive interaction can produce tension but also leads to new directions and improvement. Positive, pleasant interaction without strong emphasis on effectiveness, like conflict without improvement, can be counterproductive.

The manager plays a key role in influencing the human climate of an organization. If the employees feel that their work is important and if their needs and goals are taken into consideration, employee morale and work output will be high.

In order to foster a positive, effective human climate, the manager needs to understand himself as a leader. He needs to be aware of his motivation and attitudes and his perception of people. With this knowledge, the manager can encourage a positive human relations program based on respect and appreciation of the employee and a sensitivity to his needs and aspirations both as an individual and as a member of a group.

THE MANAGER UNDERSTANDS HIS LEADERSHIP ROLE

To be successful in interpersonal relationships at work, the manager must be an effective leader. To make leadership a reality, the manager needs to develop personal qualities, abilities, and attitudes that produce positive relationships with the employees, other departments, the public, patients, and those in higher management circles. The manager also has to be aware of his particular leadership style. His attitudes should be based on a day-to-day sense of accountability, the ability to see things through and get things done, and the willingness to take on greater responsibility.

POST-TEST 11–1

1. List the four personal qualifications for leadership.
2. List the personal qualifications and attitudes necessary to the following department heads:
   a. Director of nursing service
   b. Director of buildings and grounds
      (i) Which personal characteristics are the same for each department head?
      (ii) Which personal characteristics are different? Why?
3. Are leadership attitudes the same for all department heads? Why?

Leadership Style

As the appointed leader of the employee group, the manager possesses certain prerogatives and authority. The way that he uses this power affects the freedom of the employees in the group productivity. As the manager exerts less authority, the group members gain greater freedom in decision making; as he displays more power, the freedom of the group declines. This relationship is shown in Figure 24.

The figure relates different kinds of leadership styles to different balances of power between the manager and his employees. Behavior at the left side of the scale can be called leader-dominated, because the decision making is based on rules and policies and strongly influenced by the leader's analysis of work problems. The behavior on the right side of the scale can be referred to as group dominated, because the decision making reflects the group members' assessment of the problem and their interests and goals.

LEADER-DOMINATED RULE-CENTERED STYLES

Autocratic and authoritarian leaders place emphasis on autonomous decision making and the importance of the rules and the work of the institution.

Autocratic.   This leader identifies a problem, gathers information about it, chooses a solution from among several alternatives, and then tells his employees what to do. He may or may not consider what he believes his employees will think or feel about this decision, but they are not allowed to participate in the decision making.

Authoritarian.   This leader also makes decisions without consulting his employees. However, instead of just announcing his decisions, he tries to explain to the employees the basis for such decisions, encourages and answers all their quetions, and supports the need for compliance.

Leaders who use these two styles of behavior stress the rules, policies, and procedures of an organization. The importance of the work is also paramount, with quality and efficiency major goals to be attained. These

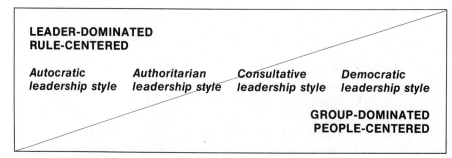

Figure 24   Continuum of leadership styles.

leaders are impersonal and formal with their employees and manifest little skill in dealing with individuals or groups.

GROUP-DOMINATED PEOPLE-CENTERED STYLES

Consultative and democratic leaders place emphasis on the employees' involvement in the decision making and the maintenance of a cohesive group spirit.

Consultative. This leader gives the employees a chance to influence the decision making from the beginning. He presents the problem, asks for employee feedback on how to solve it, and then selects the most appropriate solution.

Democratic. This leader participates in the discussion as a member of the group and agrees to carry out the group's decision.

Leaders using these two behavior patterns focus on the person and the group. Work is accomplished through individuals, with team spirit stressed continually. Employees working with these leaders receive encouragement to develop their abilities and assume greater responsibilities.

Naturally, very few managers conform exactly to any one of these patterns. Most people remain somewhat flexible in their approach to different situations, and often the leadership style of a middle manager is greatly influenced by the behavior of top management. However, most supervisors tend to focus on one or another of these styles when they direct the work of others. Furthermore, there are situations in which each of these patterns of leadership is more efficient and appropriate than the others.

In some situations, autonomous decision-making produces the best results, with rules and policies adhered to exactly. For example, in an emergency situation, such as a fire in the building, speed of action determines success. There is no time to obtain a group consensus on the best course of action. One person must decide what shall be done. In another instance, safety may necessitate that procedures concerned with the installation of new equipment or an accident on the job be followed closely.

On the other hand, involvement of the employees in deciding future plans for the department does aid in the implementation of the plans. Group decision-making is also successful when members of the group are professionals, have equal information or each possess some unique specialized knowledge about a problem, and can exercise independent judgment. A case in point would be the laboratory technologists deciding on the best procedure for doing an SMA 12 profile.

There are also advantages and disadvantages to each style of leadership. Under the autocratic and authoritarian styles, the employees lack opportunities to use their initiative. As a result, they may become frustrated and fail to produce quality work. However, these rule-centered styles simplify methods for getting the work done. Also, the rules and procedures are closely followed, since the communication and directives come from the top down.

The advantages of the consultative-participative and democratic styles of leadership revolve around the meaningful involvement of the workers, which greatly facilitates the implementation of the decisions that have been made. The disadvantages of these approaches are related to longer time needed to make decisions. Also, when the democratic forms of leadership are used, the leader can lose control of the work force if the group is allowed complete autonomy.

In summary, the effective leader is flexible in his behavior and chooses from a range of leadership styles, depending upon the situation. He is further aware of the forces within himself, the group, and the environment, and he chooses his leadership style after assessing these factors. Regardless of his style, the effective leader should strive to maintain the quality of the work, raise employee morale, and assist the institution in developing a responsiveness to change.

POST-TEST 11–2

Mr. Stevens was promoted to the position of acting director of housekeeping after the sudden death of Mr. Hall, who had been the department head for 10 years. Mr. Stevens, who had been an area housekeeping supervisor, knew that if he did a good job, the promotion would be permanent; otherwise, another department head would be recruited. After deciding that too much time had been spent previously on departmental meetings and employee conferences, Mr. Stevens called all the employees together and told them that the weekly departmental meetings were canceled, and changes in procedures would be decided by him and communicated in memos. In keeping with his policy of absolute control, Mr. Stevens failed to support his subordinates when complaints arose about their work and often spoke ill of them to Mr. Glaser, the assistant administrator. One day the hospital basement flooded. Most of the housekeeping employees ignored the situation and continued their routine tasks. Mr. Stevens was not there because he had taken the afternoon off without telling anyone.

1. Which leadership style does Mr. Stevens approximate?
2. Discuss the behavior of Mr. Stevens in relation to
   a. employee morale
   b. work output of the housekeeping department
   c. quality of work of the housekeeping employees
3. What leadership qualities should Mr. Stevens develop?

THE MANAGER UNDERSTANDS THE EMPLOYEE

Besides developing sensitivity to his role as a leader, the manager must also appreciate his employees as unique individuals and as members of a group.

The life view that the employee brings to the work situation is a combination of his individual needs, motivations, hereditary traits, and environmental influences. The employee also has a particular set of physical and mental abilities.

Hereditary and Environmental Factors

Every person is similar in his need for physical and emotional satisfaction. Everyone must breathe, eat, and sleep. Furthermore, everyone needs affection, close relationships, and acceptance by others. However, the extent to which a person manifests these needs varies according to his hereditary background, environment, and physical and mental characteristics.

Differences among people are strongly influenced by hereditary and environmental factors. Heredity influences physical characteristics such as appearance, height, and strength; it also affects personality development and sets certain boundaries to one's mental ability.

Concomitantly, environmental factors play a critical role in the development of the individual. These factors encompass all the events that happen to an individual in his lifetime. Through life experiences, the person takes on his own interests, attitudes, skills, knowledge, and a unique personality structure. The experiences in a person's environment include those dealing with his family, work, and recreation.

Physical and Mental Factors

Each individual employee brings to his job singular physical and mental characteristics.

PHYSICAL FACTORS

Physical characteristics are genetically determined and are defined at birth. However, certain environmental factors play an important role in a person's physical development. Where and how a person grew up and what he ate and how active he was also have a great bearing on his physical capacities.

Hence, the state of a person's health plays an important role in work efficiency. For example, a nurse's aide who grew up in a crowded urban area and on an improper diet might be physically weaker than her friend who was raised on a farm and always received fresh vegetables and plenty of milk and eggs. The person who has physical and mental disequilibrium does not have the energy to perform satisfactorily at work. As a result he may frequently be absent from work because of sickness.

The importance of other physical factors varies with the particular job. For example, the machine processing of vouchers in the business office requires special physical qualifications; assisting in surgery requires highly developed coordination and motor ability.

If people are physically suited to their jobs, they will be happier and more efficient, there will be greater productivity, and the morale will be high. If a person lacks the physical capability to perform a particular job, more frequent accidents, absenteeism, high turnover, and dissatisfaction may result.

MENTAL FACTORS

Although heredity plays an important part in determining a person's basic mental endowments, many environmental factors determine whether he develops his mental abilities to the fullest. A worker needs to be suited to his job in terms of intelligence, aptitude, knowledge, and skills.

Intelligence is an overall potential for understanding, reasoning, remembering, problem solving, and conceptual thinking. A person with a low IQ may not be able to grasp the variables of a difficult management problem or of a complex social or patient-care situation.

Aptitude, on the other hand, is a potential in a particular area. One person in a department might have an aptitude for fixing machines; another might have an aptitude for organizing and directing people.

The mental skills needed for each job in the institution should be delineated. For example, the director of nursing services must solve complicated human-relations and organizational problems, while the worker on the tray line has to be able to understand the flow of the trays as they are assembled. Prospective employees should be tested to determine their intelligence and aptitude to perform the job for which they are applying.

POST-TEST 11–3

1. List the four factors that make each employee a unique individual.

2. List the physical and mental qualifications for the following positions:

Position	Physical Qualifications	Mental Qualifications
Switchboard operator		
Hospital administrator		
Keypunch operator		
Registered nurse—intensive care		

THE MANAGER UNDERSTANDS THE GROUP PROCESS

Most people are members of many groups: the family, church committees, bridge clubs, bowling leagues, unions, discussion groups, and university classes. However, one of the most influential group structures is the work unit, a collection of people responsible for certain functions within an organization who interact on multiple social levels with each other. The effective manager understands the structure and functioning of the various work groups, the role of the individual employee within each group, and the efficient use of group effort.

Types of Groups

There are two kinds of groups in the work environment—the formal and the informal.

Formal groups are those determined by the organizational structure. These groups have a definite function, organization, and membership. For example, the inhalation therapy department of a 400-bed hospital is a formal organizational entity, the purpose of which is to provide therapeutic gases to patients with respiratory conditions. It is organized under the direction of a chief therapist functioning as the department head, with inhalation therapists and aides reporting to him. Personnel in the department are specially trained and certified to carry out specified functions, and they interact in a certain way with the patients and other professional employees.

Informal groups, on the other hand, develop around common interests and needs of people. Those within the group reflect similar values, motivations, and a feeling of fellowship for each other. Informal groups develop to play baseball, enjoy lunch, and discuss new books. These groups usually cut across departmental lines and organizational levels in a hospital. Examples of these groups are the bowling team formed by the pharmacy and physical therapy employees, and the maintenance and housekeeping employees who have their coffee breaks together.

The importance of a manager's understanding of the objectives and interaction of formal and informal groups cannot be overstressed. In formal groups, certain behaviors flow from the function of the group, the policies governing the department, and the expectations of others toward this department. Informal groups are more spontaneous in their development and organization. However, they are no less important to the smooth functioning of an organization, because they can aid a manager in obtaining the cooperation of a large employee unit and building a team spirit.

Every group has its own dynamics; that is, its members interact in a certain manner so that the behavior of the group is predictable. The process that occurs as group members interact influences the product of the group. In the institutional setting, this would be the work itself.

A quality product from a group depends chiefly on the involvement of the group members in the decision-making process. This means that members of the group should be encouraged to voice their opinions and offer solutions to problems encountered in the work environment. Since the group assumes its own personality, it can go about its activities in a mature fashion or dissipate its energies in destructive or non–work-oriented behavior.

Groups may be encouraged to develop in positive directions through coaching, reinforcement, and the accountability of progress toward goals. Finally, a group becomes more cohesive and productive as its members assume responsibility for the way the group acts.

POST-TEST 11–4

1. Define the two kinds of work groups.
2. Check the appropriate column for each of the following groups:

	Formal Group	Informal Group
Directors of clinical laboratories		
Memorial Hospital		
3E bowling league		
Memorial hospital employees' picnic		
Pleasantville Comprehensive Health Planning Agency		

Importance of the Group for the Individual

The work group influences a person's behavior, motivation, attitudes, and frustration level. If a work group achieves cohesion and mutually reinforcing behavior, employees will be more likely to have high morale and a sense of accomplishment and to take pride in the quality of their work. Conversely, tension among some or all members of a group makes them feel less than welcome. Friction often develops, manifesting itself in high turnover, absenteeism, accidents, and lowered productivity.

In order for work groups to function effectively, the needs of the individual within the group must be recognized and met. The employee wants to belong to both the formal and informal units of the organization. As a result, he needs to feel that he is welcome and that no one objects to his presence. He wants to have something to say about the goals adopted by the group and about what will be expected of him to carry out these goals. Finally, the employee needs to be kept informed of the progress of the group in attaining the established goals.

POST-TEST 11–5

Discuss why the group is important for the individual employee.

Facilitation of Group Effort

To facilitate the efficient operation of the group, the manager needs to perform certain activities related to the tasks assigned to the group and to maintenance of group cohesiveness. These functions are described in the following paragraphs.

TASK FUNCTIONS

Initiating and proposing goals—suggesting an idea for the solution of a problem or proposing objectives that can be adopted by the group.

Miss Hund, head nurse on Ward 1W, suggests that laundry packs be passed out by the ward secretary so that the nursing staff can begin to give patients their morning care sooner.

Information-getting—seeking relevant facts for the solution of a problem.

Prior to a meeting of all the dietary department employees, Mr. Higgins talks to the food service managers in four other hospitals to determine how other dietary departments keep the patients' food hot.

Information-giving—providing relevant facts to the group so that they can solve problems and formulate goals more easily.

Miss Jones, the director of the business office, tells her employees about the new policy on overtime payment.

Clarifying—clearing up confusion by sharing ideas, suggestions, policies, and procedures.

In a meeting of the employees of the medical records department, Mr. Arnold, the chief record librarian, cites the advantages and disadvantages of initiating a central dictating system for medical records.

MAINTENANCE FUNCTIONS

Encouraging—being friendly, warm, and open to the employees as a group so they will feel they are accepted and contributing to the group goals.

Mr. Westers, the director of purchasing, asks each of his employees about their families as he visits the stockroom.

Harmonizing—attempting to reduce tension due to disagreements and friction between members of the group.

Two employees who disagree on methods of transporting patients from the admitting office to the nursery ward are asked to discuss their ideas with Mr. Rogers, the director of the admissions department.

Setting standards — defining standards for work performances.

Mr. Bourke, the chief laboratory technologist, discusses with the other technologists the optimal turnaround time for a complete blood count.

All groups, regardless of size or purpose, need task and maintenance activity. The most effective groups are those in which the members assume responsibility for these functions rather than having the manager alone perform them. However, the manager must create an environment in which these activities are constantly evident.

POST-TEST 11–6

List four ways in which the manager can facilitate group effort.

THE MANAGER UNDERSTANDS POSITIVE HUMAN RELATIONS

Successful human relations implies a *positive* regard for others and a climate of development within the organization.

Positive Regard for People and Enhancement of Self-Esteem

Positive regard for others occurs when a person's self-esteem is enhanced and he is accepted and approved. People respond positively when their self-esteem is enhanced. Employees produce superior work when they know they are approved of and accepted by their fellow workers and supervisors. Every person wants to grow in his job and contribute to the organization for which he works. He needs approval of others so he can approve of himself — in other words, when a person feels good about himself, he'll feel good about others. When self-esteem is damaged, friction and tension with others result.

ACCEPTANCE

When a person is accepted, he is received favorably without having his behavior judged. It is difficult not to evaluate others; external judgment occurs constantly in daily living. Such phrases as "That's good!"

"That's horrible!" and "That shouldn't be!" are familiar to everyone. Evaluations of this type force the individual to defend his behavior when he would prefer simply to modify his actions to achieve better results.

If the manager can keep the relationship with the employee free of judgment, the individual will recognize that the locus of responsibility for his actions lies within himself, not with other people in his environment. He will also feel free to be himself around his supervisor, since he is accepted and respected as a worthwhile person.

Acceptance, then, implies that the manager has a positive regard for the person, that he shows him respect and understands that the employee has his own feelings and expresses them in his own way. This attitude helps the individual employee to develop his personality and manifest his talents without fear of rejection and disapproval.

APPROVAL

Approval implies the confirmation of the person by his peers and supervisors. The person is appreciated and noticed for who he is and what he is contributing to the institution. This attitude is shown by being courteous and considerate of the individual employee, by being on time for appointments, calling him by name, and giving credit for suggestions he makes.

Acceptance and approval of others facilitate positive human relationships. When people feel appreciated, they are happier and want to do a better job. These positive attitudes about others can be developed by realizing that other people are important, by noticing other people, and by not being condescending in any way toward another person.

POST-TEST 11–7

1. List three ways that a manager can show positive regard for other people.

2. June Adams had just finished feeding Mrs. Stone, a patient on the rehabilitation unit, when Mrs. Glaver, RN, the team leader, came into the room and said in a loud voice, "Mrs. Adams, I have lost all patience with you. How many times do I have to remind you that the 11 o'clock temperatures are to be turned in before the lunch trays arrive? Because of your irresponsibility, Dr. Ganen is upset that he wasn't notified sooner about his patient's elevated temperature."

Miss Adams starts to cry and runs to the utility room, where she tells three other nurse's aides that "Mrs. Glaver is the meanest woman I have ever worked with."

Discuss how this situation could have been handled by Mrs. Glaver so that Miss Adams's self-esteem would have been maintained.

3. Thank an employee for a good job in the presence of another person.

4. Listen with an open mind to a person with an opposing view on politics.

Climate of Development

One of the important reasons that people become affiliated with an institution is to develop additional knowledge and skills through their work experience. They look to the institution to facilitate their self-actualization.

A non-punishing and friendly environment aids the development of the individual. If he feels that he is needed and trusted, he will be motivated to perform better on his job and often will ask for additional responsibilities. Furthermore, employees grow when they have something to say about the organization of their own work. If a laundry worker has his own routine for loading and unloading the extractor, he should be allowed to do the activity as he wishes. Likewise, if he wants to experiment with a different procedure, he should be given the encouragement and freedom to try different methods.

Probably the most effective development of people is through day-to-day contact with the supervisor. Each meeting with the employee is an opportunity for the supervisor to help him grow and develop. The manager, through his good example, can demonstrate a sense of integrity and inspire confidence in his workers. When an employee agrees to development on his job, he weighs the investment against the sincerity and honesty of his supervisor. If he does not trust the supervisor, he will go through the motions of improvement, but he will not develop.

On-the-job contacts further insure that the employee understands his job, that his performance is evaluated, and feedback is given so that he can organize a program of improvement if necessary.

Managers should know their employees well enough so that an individualized program of development can be fashioned for each worker. This development plan should take into account the previous educational and work experience of the employee, with a view to the development of the knowledge and skills to help him progress in his work.

POST-TEST 11–8

Discuss two ways that a manager can facilitate a climate of development for his employees.

SUMMARY

Positive human relationships are one of the most essential elements of a productive work situation. Employees and supervisors need to feel that they are accepted and respected as unique individuals who are trying to make a worthwhile contribution to a collective task.

The manager plays a key role in creating a positive human climate through understanding his own and other leadership styles, by being sensitive to each of his employees as individuals, and through facilitating the group process in a positive way. If people in the work environment feel that they are contributing to a major effort, they will grow and support the organization.

RECAP EXERCISE II

Ms. Mary Peters, the laboratory supervisor, is responsible for 75 employees and 6 clinical supervisors. She likes her job, and the supervisors and employees who work for her cooperate with her in every way.

This morning when she came to work, she noticed that one of her clinical supervisors, Bill Thompson, was late in getting to work. Since Bill is very conscientious and was setting up new procedures for hematological tests, Ms. Peters wondered what had happened. Bill is thoroughly dependable and always calls when he is going to be detained. For this reason, Ms. Peters was concerned and was about to call his home when one of Bill's men, a technician named Henry Black, came in. Henry, a good-natured youth, just out of junior college, is obviously angry and tells Ms. Peters he is not going to work for Bill another minute and will quit unless he can have another job. It seems that Bill did come in, started to work, and then lost his temper when young Henry didn't do something quite right.

Mary is aware that occasionally Bill has bad moods. However, he seldom loses his temper around the employees. The responsibility for changing all of the hematology procedures may have put him under too much pressure, but even so, his outburst this morning seems difficult to explain on any reasonable grounds. Ms. Peters feels that there is something seriously wrong and that if she can get Bill to talk about what is bothering him, she can straighten out the situation.

After she talked with Henry for several minutes, he felt better and was ready to go back on the job. Ms. Peters telephoned Bill and asked him to drop around when he had a chance. Bill said he would come right over and is walking towards Ms. Peters's office now.

1. Delineate some of the human-relations problems in this situation.

2. Based on the principles enumerated in the chapter, what considerations should Ms. Peters think through before talking with Bill Thompson?

3. If you were Ms. Peters, how would you handle this situation?

REFERENCES

1. Alderfer, Clayton P.: *Existence, Relatedness and Growth: Human Needs in Organizational Settings.* New York, The Free Press, 1971.
2. Argyris, C.: *Interpersonal Competence and Organizational Effectiveness.* Homewood, Ill., Irwin-Dorsey, 1962.
3. Beach, D.: *The Management of People at Work.* New York, Macmillan, Inc., 1967.
4. Bennis, Warren G.: *Changing Organizations.* New York, McGraw-Hill Book Co., 1968.
5. Davis, Keith: *Human Relations at Work: The Dynamics of Organizational Behavior,* 3rd ed. New York, McGraw-Hill Book Co., 1967.
6. Kiesler, C. A., Collins, B. E., and Miller, N.: *Attitude Change.* New York, John Wiley & Sons, Inc., 1969.
7. Likert, R.: *The Human Organization.* New York, McGraw-Hill Book Co., 1967.
8. McGregor, D.: *The Human Side of Enterprise.* New York, McGraw-Hill Book Co., 1960.
9. Morris, Jud: *The Art of Listening.* Boston, Cahners Publishing Co., 1971.
10. Reeves, Elton T.: *The Dynamics of Group Behavior.* New York, American Management Association, 1970.
11. Triggs, Thomas, and Pickett, Ronald: *Human Factors in Health Care.* Lexington, Mass., D. C. Heath & Co., 1975.

CONSIDERATIONS FOR CONTINUING EDUCATION IN MANAGEMENT: EPILOGUE AND PROLOGUE

INTRODUCTION

During the past few years, criticism of the health care delivery system has grown to encompass the issues of both efficiency and effectiveness. People outside and inside the system express dissatisfaction at such things as allowing wards with unneeded bed capacity to be built, failure to control costs of operation through effective manpower utilization, and concentrating on high-cost procedures of unproven value. Unionization of employees has grown partly as a result of failures to develop management skills and work systems.

Not all of the tools necessary to cope with such problems have been covered in this text, but many of use in the day-to-day management of human resources have been described. Is the need for such skills and knowledge likely to be more or less important in the future? Should mastering the material covered here be necessary and sufficient, or will further work be required? Our answer is that concepts, methods, and skills covered here will become increasingly important and that this work can represent a start but not the endpoint of one's development.

SOCIETAL TRENDS: INPUTS TO HEALTH SERVICE SYSTEMS

Our society continues to urbanize, bringing more people into smaller and smaller spaces. Compactness increases the need for tighter organization and greater complexity of all services, including health care. It also

209

encourages greater specialization of resources — a trend noticed in medical education during the past few decades.

Along with more compact communities, mobility increases steadily. Two- and three-car families using crowded freeways face greater risk of trauma, a situation currently receiving greater attention with the development of specialized trauma centers and the training and deployment of paramedics. Occupational and social mobility continue to increase as educational levels rise and opportunities for specialization increase.

In spite of periodic downturns, affluence among the population spurs consumer industry growth, including health care services. Such affluence, coupled with higher levels of education and instant media reporting on new treatments and "cures," increases pressures for having more of everything available in every health center (hospital, doctor's office, and corner drugstore). This pressure for the latest advances affects many decision processes, often leading to the overstocking of some very expensive technology, which in turn increases the cost to the consumer.

Consumerism and a focus upon discrimination and rights grow in importance. Equality for minorities, for women, and for the poor all undergird the push for health as a right. The desire for equal rights has recently been backed up with pressure to finance the rights involved. Medicaid, Medicare, and other programs that will follow provide funds to those not previously enjoying sufficient purchasing power to secure services on the same basis as the more affluent. The involvement of more federal funds provides leverage for minorities and women to gain greater recognition from health care employers for their aspirations for upward job mobility and education. Education and television coverage also fuel the drive for rights and the implementation of such rights through organizational changes and financing of necessary programs. This trend seems likely to continue.

Major infectious diseases and acute care problems seem to be largely under control. Many of the precursors of today's killers appear to be outside the traditional range of medical practice until they reach an acute stage. Heart disease, obesity, alcoholism, and other serious conditions appear to require life-style modification, an area of individual and social choice. The conditions leading to such problems and their "cure" change slowly and over long periods of time, making them seem to be outside the realm of an acute-care oriented system of medical services. Chronic illness and maintenance of persons with disability rise in prominence as the population ages and the aged constitute a larger proportion of the total population. Critics of the current system abound, and many thoughtful people on all sides of the issues wonder whether a major shift in our approach to servicing human needs must be implemented.

Many changes in our society point to the need for more creative responses from the health care system. In addition, effective demands for health care will increase — demands that will be backed with money.

IMPLICATIONS OF SOCIETAL CHANGE FOR THE HEALTH FIELD

Movement from emphasis on acute care to ambulatory care of preventive medicine will occur. More clinics and diagnostic centers will be developed close to consumers. Prepayment plans, group practice, "health maintenance organizations," and other forms of health care organizations will emerge. New forms of health manpower, similar to physician assistants, nurse practitioners, and emergency medical technicians, will be developed.

Hospitals and other health care facilities will need to be expanded and modernized, with due attention given to the heavy population growth areas in the nation's suburbs. Cost factors, including the heavy duplication of high-cost technology and beds, will result in stronger consumer and governmental pressure to control expansion and growth. Regional planning, rate controls, franchising of new operations, and specialized care centers will grow in importance. Recently, national health planning legislation stressed the need for stronger planning and resource allocation. The national priorities stressed in this legislation emphasize management of systems containing all levels of care.

Planning and resource allocation programs mandated earlier will provide a base for the development of sounder, more thorough control systems than have existed in the past. New legislation extending federally financed or guaranteed health care benefits to larger segments of the population seems inevitable. Given the incremental fashion in which our pluralistic system operates, however, the enterprising manager is assured of an opportunity and a responsibility to continue to come up with creative solutions to problems. Magic answers and national solutions to local problems are nonexistent.

LONG-RANGE MANAGEMENT CONSIDERATIONS

The changes noted above should be incorporated into one's thinking when considering long-range planning. Are any of your plans likely to be subject to the approval of planning agencies? Is the local school system, college, or other such organization likely to supply you with manpower in the future? Are any of your clinical programs likely to shift because of new funding, changes in disease patterns, or age composition of the population served?

In looking at how you currently organize your work and perform various tasks, do you anticipate some technological innovation to replace old procedures? Remember that as labor becomes more expensive (increased skills, education base, and unionization) it is possible to seek and usually to find substitutions. With cost continuing to rise, can some of your expenses, such as those for entry education, be shifted to other parts of the community? The search for alternatives must continue unabated as the pressures for more effective management continue to increase.

THE MANAGEMENT RESPONSE

Throughout this book, the management response has been stressed. Conceptual models, technical skills, and human skills are the tools that managers use to think about their work and to fashion solutions to old and new problems.

We work and live with systems every day. Inputs, throughputs, and outcomes are mentally manipulated constantly to see whether alternatives can be devised to help us perform more effectively. Problems of production, adaptation, maintenance, and governance recur daily and need attention. Scheduling, planning, personal appraisal, and control systems require constant monitoring to insure appropriate functioning.

Managers must sift through the welter of activity and events to find the most appropriate focus for their strategy and planning activities. In a dynamic society and workplace, it is very easy to miss the important issues amid the daily routines that constantly demand attention. Effective managers invariably are those who recognize the important, fundamental, and lasting elements and act on them.

Motivating of employees and superiors, communicating, and understanding the necessary exchanges that make up social life constitute important skills that must be continually honed and developed in order to insure that productivity flows through the proper channels. A strategy without a plan, like a plan without a following, does very little for anyone. Implementation without controls or without a target may or may not succeed. In any event, no one will know, since no one knows where you are trying to go in the first instance. The output from a sound management approach will be a soundly managed operation; and neither can be achieved if you do not have the necessary skills for the job.

The management response to health systems should result in more cost-effective care, appropriate to needs and accessible to the population. The external pressure to move in this direction exists and increasingly employers look to their management staffs to cut cost and improve controls and effectiveness and to do so with the same or a lower budget than before. This does not rule out new investments or even higher cost for some activities, but the days when costs did not even get serious consideration have passed.

CONTINUING EDUCATION

Anyone who has stayed with us throughout this exercise already has a sound basis for continuing their education in management. Articles and books on the subject abound and can be found in every major library and in almost all of the professional journals in the field. All one needs to do to gain major benefit from such material is to subject them to the test of appropriateness in your own area of work. Pick out the key ideas and use them to take inventory of your own practices and performance. Design your own exercises, using facts and situations that you face every day.

On any given day, in almost every city in the country, one can find some type of management development course or associated program with management implications to attend. High schools, night schools, community colleges, and others offer an abundance of courses on a variety of related topics. Most employers would be more than happy to respond positively to supervisor request for more management training either on or off the job.

REFERENCES

1. American College of Hospital Administrators: *National Health Insurance: Principles of a Successful Program.* Chicago, American College of Hospital Administrators, 1974.
2. American Hospital Association: *Quality Assurance Program for Medical Care in the Hospital.* Chicago, American Hospital Association, 1972.
3. Bryant, John: *Health and the Developing World.* Ithaca, N. Y., Cornell University Press, 1969.
4. Cowen, D. L., and Sharbaro, J. A.: Timely-centered health care: A viable reality? *Med. Care 10*:164–172, March–April, 1972.
5. Drucker, Peter T.: *The Age of Discontinuity.* New York, Harper and Row, 1969.
6. Goble, Frank: *Excellence in Leadership.* New York, American Management Association, 1972.
7. Kahn, Herman (ed.): *The Future of the Corporation.* New York, Mason and Lipscomb, 1974.
8. Kissick, William L.: Health policy directions for the 1970's. *N. Engl. J. Med. 282*:1343–1354, 1970.
9. McGregor, Douglas: *The Professional Manager.* New York, McGraw-Hill Book Co., 1967.
10. Schein, Edgar: *Professional Education.* New York, McGraw-Hill Book Co., 1971.
11. Somers, Anne R.: *Health Care in Transition: Directions for the Future.* Chicago, Hospital Research and Educational Trust, 1971.

Selected Readings

INTRODUCTION

Modern health care and business organizations must deal with change in the internal operating arena and in the larger community. Changes requiring the redesign of organizations include new professions, new technology, new services such as ambulatory, chemical addiction, and health education programs. At the larger system level health care institutions are being asked to share programs, merge, build satellites, deliver all levels of care, and operate in new and changing communities. Luke's article deals with the major theories and approaches to designing organizations and managing the fit between individuals and organizations. Brown and Money deal primarily with major changes obscuring in the organization and management of hospitals and other health care organizations, namely the movement to large scale systems of hospitals.

Luke stresses the interface between individuals and their own organization imbedded in the fabric of individual circumstance. He points out the major approaches designed to assist in the organizational change process. Finally he presents an idea that managers themselves should be change agents. Many of the concepts and theories presented here underlie the development of this book and the suggestion that managers themselves can become major leaders in the organizational renewal and change.

Exercise

1. Consider the major assumptions about how man and organizations behave and list the assumptions about people held by managers in your organization.
2. Consider the model of man which you feel best fits the behavior of people in your organization.
3. List the major and minor changes which you feel should be made to help your organization improve the fit between the organization and the individuals.

Brown and Money provide an overview of the ways in which individual hospitals are moving into shared services and into systems of hospitals. These new organizations have the size to afford many more types of management specialties than one can afford in a single organization. More organizations are sharing certain types of personnel, developing joint ventures, and specializing in programs.

Exercise

1. Consider the implications of this type of change for your own organization.
2. What types of services might you specialize in, and what would you suggest that other neighboring institutions provide?
3. What parts of your own area of responsibility would be enhanced if you were linked into other such service programs with other institutions?
4. If you were personally responsible for your own type of activity in five institutions instead of one, what would be the implications for your own level of educational and experimental requirements?
5. Would people handling the individual five programs need the same level of competence as yourself, or could someone with less preparation handle the job?
6. If your organization considered contracting to manage another similar organization, would you benefit from providing consultation in your own area of expertise?
7. What kind of economies would be likely to result from such sharing?
8. What kinds of "people problems" would you anticipate?
9. What types of reward systems would be needed to get full cooperation in the new organization?
10. What types of educational programs would be needed to prepare people for new roles and responsibilities?

In summary, there is a new world of organizations that is changing the roles and responsibilities of managers in health care. It is exciting, but it will require all our creative talents and energies to make it work. More questions could be asked than answered—but that is the nature of dynamic organizations.

The Promise of Multihospital Management*

Montague Brown, DPH, and William H. Money

One decade ago at Duke University the late Ray Brown chaired the First National Forum on Hospital and Health Affairs whose topic was "Multiple Hospital Units Under Single Management." Brown pointed out that community hospitals, confronted with increasing pressures for greater efficiency and reduced cost, could more easily solve their problems by joining together. At the same time, other participants advocated the perpetuation of autonomous community hospitals and pressed for concentrating hospital efforts on meeting the needs and desires of the present users of service and not on further development. During this early discussion, some of the advantages and disadvantages of multiple unit systems surfaced while the participants analyzed why these organizations were developing.

Urban sprawl with its attendant population shifts clearly helped to spur development of the branch or satellite hospital whose benefits included lower capital outlay, easy access to a "mother" hospital, an established medical staff, and preexistent administrative expertise. Mergers occurred between hospitals caught in financial binds as their communities found themselves less able to afford the services offered. Planning agencies, although relatively disorganized and weak at this point, favored a more rational allocation of care provided among competing hospitals and recommended mergers and shared services.

Other participants in that first Duke Forum predicted that multiple units, especially in the more prosperous communities, would prove neither feasible nor a major force in the organization of hospitals in the future. But systems seem to have become more feasible and desirable during the 10 years since the Duke Forum first debated this strategy for organizing and delivering health care.

"SYSTEMATIZING" CATHOLIC HOSPITALS

The multiple unit management system is indeed an important issue for Catholic hospitals. In 1970, after several years of study, the Catholic Hospital Association developed the Catholic Health Services Leadership Program (CHSLP). The program explicitly recognizes the

---

*Hosp. Progr. 56:36–42, 1975.

strength and advantages of a corporate, multiple-unit hospital system and the need for decentralized management of the local hospital. Furthermore, the program recognizes the capacity of Catholic-owned groups of hospitals to literally and figuratively alter the health service delivery systems of this country by making their hospital operations more systematic by employing the multiple-unit management strategy.

If only a small percentage of the current cost of operating relatively autonomous individual hospitals could be saved by this strategy, sufficient resources would be available to support the Church's missionary work in other aspects of public health. Catholic health care institutions have the economic capacity, the Christian mission, and the organization and resolve to provide leadership. Certainly, the health care field today needs such leadership. Will the Catholic health care community respond?

Others are in a position to provide leadership in health care delivery, but their availability neither absolves the Catholic community from responsibility nor mitigates its opportunity to benefit mankind by accepting a leadership role. Catholic input can insure the integration of Christian compassion and sound management strategy into a national health service system that includes Catholic community hospitals.

What led to the Duke Forum prediction which has been wrong for at least a decade? The advantages of economies of scale were perceived as relating to shared services, purchasing, blood banks, maintenance and repair, data processing, laundry, and specialized equipment. The disadvantages were related to provincial self-interest, possible excessive standby cost associated with multiple units (where excess beds and services prevailed), staffing problems, and difficulties in getting uniform policies.

Both the advantages and disadvantages still are present in today's systems, and were we simply to use these factors to analyze the potential growth of systems, we would reach similar conclusions. However, these data were not the only factors which created strong pressures for the continued development of hospital systems. The health delivery industry environment for the decade 1955-65 was dramatically different from the decade now ending. Current conditions support the development of systems and have made them both a feasible and growing force in the organization of health care.

During the last 10 years, social programs promoting greater demand for health care have been developed by numerous government agencies; large sums have been spent on health-related research; building and development monies have been funneled into the health care field; and the government has moved to assess, measure, and regulate the organizations and impacts of these funds. In addition, the country experienced a period of relative boom and another of bust; the health delivery industry experienced ever-increasing public demand for more comprehensive and accessible services but at lower cost.

FORCES AFFECTING PAST SYSTEMS GROWTH

Many forces coincided to bring small and independent hospitals into more cooperative relationships.[1] First the forces favoring efficiency and cost effectiveness became more salient as government became a major purchaser of care. Highly expensive technological developments are not required in all institutions. It became futile for every hospital to attempt to remain a comprehensive island of total excellence. The third-party payers and increasingly strong planning agencies began insisting that areawide considerations of total community need take precedence over individual hospital aspirations. But who would decide what institutions would provide which services? The answer is nearly always controversial; but it is less so in a systematic operation whereby the final decision can be made by trustees who can appropriately assess financial ability and medical need while significantly reducing the amount of expensive interhospital bargaining, conflict, and competition.

The health care field's profit potential was recognized by entrepreneurs seeking additional methods of utilizing capital. The movement was developed partially through government rationalization efforts, combined with government's apparent willingness to pay for nursing homes and extended care benefits for older citizens. The government's actions lent a new impetus to the already strong position of investor-owned organizations in the long-term care field. Profit opportunities from expansion and vertical integration into the acute care market attracted investor capital and a new spirit of entrepreneurship not previously found in the autonomous voluntary community hospital. These multiple unit organizations (profit *and* nonprofit) quickly learned that advantages can accrue from *properly utilized* large-scale organization.

These special hospital organizations can realize a profit because they have certain advantages over other businesses:

1. The soundly planned hospital is almost recession proof.

2. The real estate around the hospital offers the hospital owner an advantageous investment opportunity.

3. The spreading of debt guarantees over many hospitals significantly reduces the lender's risks.

4. The benefits from indepth specialization and controls include: cash management; legal services (planning, reimbursement, malpractice); efficient land use and development; marketing and recruitment among local physicians; the expertise of a planning agency specialist who helps all units cope with the maze of regulations and power; immediate access to a labor relations expert; a hospital design specialist who is attune to economic constraints; and an engineering group which insures design appropriate to lower cost, new manpower utilization schemes, and local demand for services.

This list of benefits could be further expanded by examining the types of specialists currently used by some of the larger investor-owned nonprofit hospital chains and religious orders. Many investor and nonprofit hospital systems, as well as many larger and more sophisticated free-standing hospitals, already employ such expertise effectively and benefit greatly from doing so.

Available data is not complete, but it does indicate that the voluntary, nonprofit, free-standing (autonomous) hospital may simply be too small to make effective use of the management, technical, and legal talents available and required by modern, large-scale corporations to operate effectively and to deal with government bureaucracy. The single hospital can neither react quickly enough to poorly conceived regulations nor afford to operate at a deficit although being assured of meeting its commitments at a later date. It may not easily change its services to meet new needs, or alter its environment if it is no longer able to survive in one location. In summary, the autonomous hospital, a captive of its environment, has little flexibility or opportunity to plan and exercise control over its destiny.

FORCES AFFECTING FUTURE SYSTEMS GROWTH

Richard Johnson has predicted that current trends toward hard economic criteria and the readiness of investor-owned systems to accept this challenge to develop hard data will lead to a two-class system of hospitals. Such a system will consist of public hospitals with local tax subsidies and investor-owned hospitals which would serve the suburban and presumably more profitable market — unless the nonprofit hospitals shifted to a posture more in keeping with economic rationale and survival.[2]

This shift in posture is apparent because nonprofit hospitals are becoming more concerned with survival and with developing an economic rationale for the delivery of medical services. The 1965 prediction that hospital systems would be neither feasible nor a major force in the development of hospital organizations is contradicted by this shift in the health care delivery industry's posture. Systems (and their development) are both feasible and a major force in the organization of health care because the industry has adopted a more critical view of health care economics.

MULTIPLE HOSPITAL MANAGEMENT FEASIBILITY

The management of health care organizations by means of multiple hospital systems will affect the development of the health delivery industry in eight different ways.

First, investor-owned system growth continues today with greater attention on total contract management (which is not contingent upon ownership) of hospitals from the planning stage through operations of the completed facility. Doctor-owned operations, public hospitals, and even medical school facilities provide a market for the management expertise and full range of specialties available to the corporations. In the present tight capital market, accompanied by both inflation and recession, this avenue offers a logical systems growth opportunity. Once the core expertise is developed in a system, that expertise can be sold either to wholly owned institutions or to those owned by other entities. If such expertise cannot be easily employed over long-term periods, e.g., in hospitals of 50 beds or less, a franchise system can provide the local operator with backup and standardized packages of control systems. Such a management package was developed for home health service and is now offered by a major drug firm.

Second, voluntary, nonprofit hospitals have continued to expand their use of shared services under the same basic theory. They achieve some of the advantages of scale and specialization in increased expertise by sharing the bill with other hospitals. The fact that chains and other multiple systems use such shared services far more frequently than individual hospitals seems to indicate that the start-up, coordination, and control cost of developing this expertise frequently may outweigh its supposed advantages in the minds of a group of autonomous hospital administrators. The exception may exist when a program is undertaken by a hospital association whose business is primarily political coordination and when political advantages may accrue from the promotion of such endeavors.

A number of supra-agencies similar to the Northwestern University–McGraw Medical Center have developed to both spur shared services projects and to more rationally allocate health care delivery roles among the relatively autonomous institutions which may be loosely associated with medical schools. The trend in these agencies for economic rationality appears to be gaining ground. The economic awareness exhibited by medical centers may be attributed to a decline in support for research and referral from the increasingly autonomous suburban hospitals.

Third, the 1974 American Hospital Association *Guide to the Health Care Field* lists 162 shared service organizations sponsored by hospitals or hospital associations which seek to spread the management cost of shared service programs across several hospitals. Some of these shared service organizations are now managing future hospitals via contract arrangements.

Fourth, mergers and stronger affiliations among institutions with varying types of sponsorship in close geographic proximity with overlapping markets seem to be continuing. Financial distress and modernization requirements seem to be strong motivating factors. While inner-city hospitals face acute problems, rural hospitals in growth areas may find it more desirable to build a centrally located facility while abandoning existing facilities or altering their previous organizational roles.

Fifth, satellites or branch hospitals remain an attractive possibility for many individual hospitals. Planning agencies apparently prefer the establishment of new facilities under the aegis of existing organizations to prevent duplication and to bring existing expertise immediately to bear on new developments. Equally important, the existing hospitals need to retain the loyalty of their current medical staffs and fend off the urge of relatively autonomous staffs to develop highly specialized programs in the newer facilities in the suburbs. The new facilities, programs, and equipment could then draw the medical staff away from the older facility to the new suburban environment. This holding action may be effective in the short-run. But farsighted administrators may well plan to make the older inner-city hospital, once the "mother" hospital, a satellite of the newly developed hospital. Such transition need not be rapid or disruptive, as the development of the Memorial Hospital System in Houston, Tex., has demonstrated.

Sixth, the church-owned multiple hospital operations seem to be selecting a variety of strategic development options. The Latter Day Saints system has elected to transfer the hospitals to a centrally owned and operated nonprofit system after a relatively recent centralization of cash and investment management. The purpose of this move seems to have been to differentiate the church's missionary efforts in health delivery and health education and give the hospitals an opportunity to concentrate more fully on the delivery of hospital services. While it is too early to determine precisely how this system will evolve, indications are that a strong, capable, central management and technical staff will develop to serve local hospitals while attention also is given to maintaining and even strengthening the local inputs to the system. Expansion in the inner mountain states appears feasible and desirable.

The Catholic-owned systems are employing several health delivery strategies. Diocesan-owned-and-operated systems seem likely to follow the pattern of large city systems with mergers, satellites, and a more centralized management staff. Religious congregation-owned systems which are not so geographically restricted appear to be undergoing major reassessments of their goals and resources. Institutions which have almost exclusive monopolistic responsibility for a regional area in which the Church's position on right-to-life issues may be compromised may be phased out by sale to the respective local communities or to other groups whose basic mission would not be so compromised. In situations where the hospitals generate income which can support other endeavors of the congregation such as education and orphanages, marginal and unprofitable functions will likely be discontinued. None of the individual religious hospitals will be able to avoid the economic imperatives of today's industry without eventually going under. There is every indication that as centralization with attendant managerial, technical, and legal specialization occurs, the central organization will then bring in lay specialists to buttress the decisions of the congregation with facts and programs which insure efficient and effective use of resources.

The congregations also will consider more carefully what markets they will enter, what type of institutions and programs will be their specialty, and which agree most constructively with their religious objectives. If congregation-owned systems move aggressively, as many may, they can benefit from systems operations while maintaining and enhancing their religious mission. The congregations must have a strong position in the more economically advantaged areas because profitable suburban markets help to generate income to supply services in more economically marginal markets and poorer communities.

Seventh, medical schools and their teaching hospitals may also move more aggressively in the future. A large base of primary and secondary care centers must be either owned or closely tied to promote referral patterns necessary for the research and teaching mission of these tertiary care institutions. Some of the growth here will come from the operation of satellite hospitals and from contract management of smaller community hospitals and adjacent marginal community hospitals. The seeding of affiliated institutions with young physicians may result in physician ties conducive to referral of patients back to physicians at the teaching center.

However, much of this program seems contingent upon relations with community hospitals which do not themselves aspire to become larger comprehensive institutions. A major contradiction seems to exist in this assumption since it is difficult to imagine a medical school faculty wanting to affiliate with any institution which did not espouse and identify with its teaching and research mission. Under these circumstances, the community hospital can anticipate strong internal pressures to emulate the teaching hospital. Ownership by the teaching center may be the major option available for the achievement of these referral objectives. Simultaneously, a separately incorporated or organizationally identified division of the medical center might be established to provide contract management and other types of shared services which would reach both the community hospital aspiring to become a medical comprehensive hospital and those desiring (or designed) to remain primarily as limited service secondary care centers. Merely remaking the community hospital into a medical center model seems self-defeating for the medical center in the long-run.

Eighth, the Kaiser-Permanente Program is a key industry example of the development of multiple hospital systems. However, this unique comprehensive systems strategy integrates corporate systems management, physician groups, comprehensive prepayment medical coverage, and health care clinics to provide health care services to specific patient populations. The importance of the medical group and prepayment mechanisms are now being nationally recognized through the development of health maintenance organizations (HMOs) while the corporate structure is being developed through many multiple hospital systems. The importance of the combination of both of these approaches for the planning of health care services has not yet been fully recognized by planning and government agencies, but other multiple hospital systems are beginning to develop HMOs and promote physician groups which are critical elements of this program.

In summary, the eight developments considered here demonstrate clearly the feasibility and already strong development of the multiple hospital system, its ability to evolve under a variety of environmental pressures, its applicability in today's medical care delivery market, and its potentially dramatic future role in the delivery of health care services.

However, only one side of the feasibility issue—the hospital administrator or manager in a position to pursue this market—has been examined. What about the market itself? Will it resist the developments of multiple units, or do these units offer advantages to certain types and kinds of institutions? Will these data demonstrate that there is a real and viable demand for the multiple hospital system as a product of the management market?

MARKET REACTION

Communities desiring a hospital, boards with failing institutions, hospitals unable to attract the quality of managerial talent necessary to thrive, and public hospitals suffering from taxpayer revolt and chronic difficulties are prime targets for reorganization through merger, acquisitions, and contract management.

Communities wishing to establish a new hospital or health care delivery organization will confront pressures from planning agencies, third-party payers, and capital financing agencies to work with *existing* institutions. Nonprofit systems, including church-owned and investor-owned systems with access to capital that is elsewhere currently in short supply, will find many opportunities in each of these market categories.

While a profile of hospitals susceptible to incorporation into large multiple hospital systems has not been compiled, some of their characteristics can be inferred from existing systems. Some combination of the following characteristics seems likely: chronically low occupancy; deficit operation; rural or inner-city location; a changing clientele with increasing medical needs and a reduced ability to readily pay for these services; geographic areas that find it difficult to attract skilled (and trained) administrators and physicians; new suburbs without a well-developed social group to aggressively pursue community needs and to furnish start-up capital; new towns; hospitals under 200 beds; and older hospitals.

The recognition that such hospitals need help of course does not insure that someone should or will rush to provide assistance. Important criteria for any assisting organization will be the potential for turning the operation around or modifying its mission so an operational break-even point, if not a profit, can be achieved.

The organizations which are most likely to respond to this need and most capable of assessing the potential of the situation are those which have acquired and made available necessary managerial talent for growth and those which have developed access to capital and determined the rate of return necessary for the employment of these resources in other markets or internally within their own organizations. Many other factors may enter into the decision to operate an additional unit, but the aforementioned represent a set of bedrock considerations. The market question still remains: Are the hospitals described above in a position to make this decision?

MANAGERIAL RESPONSIBILITY TO THE MARKET

Previous development of multiple hospital systems has taken place under more favorable economic conditions and with the assumption that hospital systems will not generally manage hospitals which are not owned by the system. As financing changed, the ownership has been modified. Ownership is now conceived of as a community trust and a representation of the invested capital resources. In today's health market, the system or manager must provide an investor with an equitable return, or at least no loss, on his investment *and* the effective and responsive health care needed by the community. Nothing more is required for the investor, for he does not own the market. Nothing less than a complete health program is demanded by the community.

Multiple unit hospital systems and local communities together have developed several alternatives for establishing systems relationships with new ownership philosophy and tight monetary policies. Forms of contract management which transfer the responsibility of day-to-day management of a hospital to another party have and will continue to provide a very attractive alternative to voluntary community groups and to governments that wish to make the institution more accountable to local people and managed by another organization. In addition, contract management offers other advantages to communities. If the community has sufficient demand to generate profits, it may wish to go the contract management route to prevent resources generated in the community from being redirected to other communities or enterprises. Contract management offers flexibility when uncertainties about the future create a difficult forecasting situation and give pause to even the most optimistic planners in an economic downturn such as we are currently experiencing. But physicians who are locally oriented may resist outside domination by sources of capital and the alteration of their established methods of making operating decisions previously determined at a local level or within individual units.

Contract management will be an important force in the future of the health care industry. It represents an action program for the development of systems and a method of meeting the health care delivery demands of the public. Opportunities exist for church, nonprofit, and investor-owned companies in this growing total hospital management market.

CONTENDERS FOR EXPANDED CONTRACT MANAGEMENT

A variety of organizations have moved toward the management and leasing of hospitals on behalf of local communities. Perhaps the best known of these systems are the investor-owned organizations, the nonprofit Lutheran Hospitals and Homes Society of North Dakota, and the nonprofit Fairview Community Hospitals of Minneapolis, Minn. During the past year, there have been a variety of other entries into this market.

At least one medical school hospital has joined the ranks of the investor-managed systems. A nationally prominent hospital management consulting firm currently manages two hospitals in order to establish their profitability before returning them to a local administrator. Many of the multiple unit systems which until now owned and operated their own units have entered the market to manage other units on behalf of other owners. A major teaching hospital with a full-time staff established a division to contract manage other hospitals. One religiously owned system is considering contract management after recently establishing two new suburban units. At least one state hospital association entered a contract management agreement to salvage a hospital operation at the request of the court rather than allow a religious group to close the hospital. One astute administrator serving several small hospitals seeks to establish a management team to both handle his current group as well as to expand operations to other interested small hospitals. Finally, a shared service corporation has complete management agreements with previous customers.

There are many contrasts between management contracts and previous methods of developing multiple hospitals systems. Voluntary, nonprofit hospitals appear to move very slowly in mergers, take long periods to develop satellites, slowly develop shared services, and gradually acquire other units and new markets. They seem to find it much easier, as do the investor-owned systems, to move into management contract situations where the capital requirements are low and managerial demands are very high. For some, spreading the overhead makes it possible to acquire high-powered, specialized managerial expertise; for others it provides a profitable outlet for experts already on staff but underutilized by existing institutional requirements.

As the **Figure** indicates, time frame differences also exist. Mergers and systems groups develop for long periods, while the management contract may be brief. Hospital personnel appear to develop few of the fears associated with mergers when contracts are signed; physicians express less opposition to these arrangements; and board members retain their autonomy and control without the threats to their existence implicit in other arrangements.

Thus, this new market vehicle, contract management, spurred by the inability of investor-owned chains to get sufficient capital for expansion, seems to offer a major opportunity for voluntary nonprofit institutions to expand without new capital and to acquire and use the vast range of managerial talent so essential to modern hospital operations. As smaller systems move to develop the necessary management strength to do an outstanding job for their own hospitals, as they must, we can expect major growth in the competition for management contracts with solo and generally weaker public and private hospitals. Perhaps the end result will be a hospital market which can buy and sell specific services and programs to truly meet the changing health needs of the general public.

FIGURE: Tentative Reorganization Observations

Arrangement	Over-All Ease	Capital	Physician	Type of Commitment	Personnel	Boards
Systems Acquisition, Mergers, Development Project	Harder to accomplish	Harder to acquire	Feels threatened	Less-specified, longer-term	Fear the change	Fear a takeover
Management Contracts, Leases	Easier to accomplish	Alternative programs available	Feels less threatened	Clearly specified, shorter-term	Are less aware of change and less afraid	Remain in control

[1]Montague Brown, "Current Trends in Cooperative Ventures," *Hospitals,* June 1, 1974, pp. 40–44.
[2]Richard Johnson, "Requiem for the Nonprofit Hospital," *Modern Hospital,* February, 1974, pp. 43–46.

Matching the Individual and the Organization

Robert A. Luke, Jr.

Among the many new and diverse challenges that managers face from day to day, there is one that is constant: how to design and develop the organization so that the structure fits the nature of the work as well as the natures of the people doing the work. As with the problems that require daily attention, there are no easy procedures for dealing with this task. And no design handbooks are applicable to all organizations.

There is, however, a substantial body of research into methods of inquiry and change—developed over the years by academicians—whose basic concern is integrating the individual with the organization. That the methods have been developed by academicians does not mean that they cannot be used by managers. The academicians' lasting contribution to organizational integration may well be their methods and processes for inquiry and change rather than their findings and models. (Researchers have tended to see their models as being applicable to a far wider range of conditions than is justifiable.)

During the past 200 years, intellectuals have studied the appropriate relationship between the individual and the organization in three distinct stages. In the experimental laboratory, the researcher first developed the scientific method of study that he later applied in the action laboratory and, finally, within organizations themselves. In this article I trace the history of this study through the three stages and then discuss some approaches managers can apply to their own inquiries and design processes.

THE OBSERVERS' APPROACH

In the late eighteenth and through the mid-nineteenth centuries, intellectuals were agreed on the necessity for a planned approach to structuring relationships between individuals and organizations.[1] Their basic assumption being that man, left to his own idiosyncratic inclinations, would be his own and others' worst enemy, they shared French social scientist Claude Saint-Simon's contention that "society is essentially governed by men. In the new it will no longer be governed except by principles."

---

[1] Footnotes are listed on page 242.

These intellectuals also shared a common method of inquiry, which, simply put, was to observe the goings-on around them and then to fit their observations to their own assumptions about the nature of man and of society's needs. Using observation, conceptualization, and logic, they derived their social blueprints. But experimentation and validity testing would have to wait for the empiricists in the twentieth century. The "sages" were content with observation and theory.

The sages: Though they might seem somewhat stuffy and dusty from our perspective, these early, mainly French, writers did put their finger on what remains an unresolved tension or dialectic—that tension between the individual's need to express himself, exert self-control, and achieve recognition (what Chris Argyris calls "competence") and society's need to organize human energy into various functional tasks. The question of their day was, as it is in ours, how to handle these apparent contradictions in a society (or organization) where personal needs are viewed as being at odds with those of the collective.

Social philosophers and writers proposed various organizational ideals, each of which was intended to reduce the individual's submission to personal authority while making him part of a functioning unit. Jean Jacques Rousseau's famous corporate community was designed to satisfy man's needs for independence, equality, and freedom. Power would rest with the entire society rather than with individuals, and man would thereby be released from personal dependencies.

Claude Saint-Simon, who felt man was motivated more by material needs, proposed that men's energies be directed away from dominating each other and toward dominating nature through the development of a rational organization. Under Saint-Simon's scheme, by adapting to the organization, man would himself become rational and at the same time his and others' wealth would increase.

Charles Fourier put forth the principle of self-interest as the organizing force. Individuals in his society would assign themselves to tasks and would be able to change them periodically. Fourier's organization would reflect, rather than stifle, man's individuality; and at the same time, given the competitive drive between individuals in the same group and the drive between groups, it would allow work to be accomplished.

Emile Durkheim (who wrote as late as 1917) created a model that called for a cohesive society to be held together by the primary elements of power and authority. As private consciences were, for Durkheim, immoral and dysfunctional, the individual's proper role would be that of an organ in a society in which his conscience is subordinate to the collective's.

Hence, though disagreeing on the form organizations ought to take, these early thinkers all made the following assumptions about man's proper relationship to organizations:

1. Man needs to be controlled because, left unchecked, he destroys and oppresses himself and others.

2. Man must choose between his needs for self-direction and society's needs for collective action.

3. A society run by men ought to be replaced with a society run by principles the intellectuals could discover.

Although these writers were prolific and vociferous, they were not granted, nor perhaps did they seek, positions where they could actually influence the decision-makers of the day. Despite revolutions, wars, and depressions, limited use was made of their observations, and then only by those seeking to justify their activities. For instance, industrial leaders frequently quoted Saint-Simon to legitimize their use of child labor to achieve maximum productivity.

In comparison with the natural sciences, the social sciences have experienced both an ignoble birth and a traumatic adolescence. The rather moralistic, subjective, and nonquantifiable observations offered by the early social thinkers hardly seemed as scientific as Newton's laws of motion, which had explanatory and predictive power. Thus, in their struggle to be accepted as full members in the scientific community, social scientists began to devote considerable energy to establishing research measures and methods that would yield hard data about people and organizations. A group of new thinkers, the empiricists, sought data free from distortion—of either the researcher or the subject—that could be used to predict and explain people's attitudes and behavior.

The empiricists: Foremost among the early empiricists in applying the scientific method to the study of organizations were Fritz J. Roethlisberger, Elton Mayo, and William J. Dickson and their colleagues, who conducted the famous Hawthorne experiments in 1924.[2]

The initial intent was to measure the effect that a host of variables, such as amount of light, timing of breaks, and so forth, had on the productivity of a specially selected group of employees in a wiring room. In the process the researchers discovered that the quality and quantity of the attention management devotes to employee needs and interests are more determinant of productivity than are the physical variables in the workplace. This finding was the first research-based challenge to the notion that individual needs for achievement, recognition, and companionship are dysfunctional elements within an organization.

Soon after the Hawthorne experiments, other social scientists tried applying the scientific method to artificially created groups to identify the relationship between a group's structure and the behavior of its members.

For instance, Kurt Lewin, Ronald Lippitt, and Ralph K. White trained group leaders to play three leadership styles—democratic, autocratic, and laissez-faire—and then rotated the leaders among different groups of children making masks.[3] The researchers discovered that levels of mask production and creativity varied from group to group; in the democratic situation both were highest. In the autocratic situation, children did what they were ordered, but as soon as the leader left the room, they changed their behavior. However, in the democratic situation, children continued with their tasks whether or not the leader was present.

Besides the finding that a group member's behavior can be affected by the group leadership, the mask making and similar experiments revealed other important lessons:

1. Conscious manipulation of a group's authority structure can affect the group's behavior and output.

2. With the scientific method, man can use his intelligence and reason to affect the pattern of relationships among people in task or problem-solving groups.

3. Human behavior is greatly influenced by the environment in which men live and work, rather than by anything endemic to the nature of man, as the sages proposed.

Thus the empiricists had discovered that the human character may be more flexible than rigid. The scientific method had almost replaced conceptualization and observation as the primary mode of inquiry into relationships between individuals and organizations, and the possibility of discovering principles for designing integrative organizations was but a step away.

THE LABORATORY EXPERIMENTERS

As interest in the field of small-group dynamics continued to grow, social researchers developed a new form of inquiry—called sensitivity training, or T-groups.[4] Initiated in 1947 as an experimental vehicle through which to learn about group leadership functions, emotional dynamics, roles, decision-making styles, developmental processes, and so on, the T-group was the social scientist's first *action* laboratory. These laboratories replaced the carefully designed experiments in which the variables were manipulated according to the dictates of hypothesis with a carefully controlled set of conditions where there was no manipulation.

These conditions included the following: introducing a group of strangers to each other in an isolated setting free of contact from society, providing group leaders knowledgeable in the area of group dynamics to assist the learning process, regularly scheduling group meetings and meal and recreation times, and having group leaders adamantly refuse to assume traditional, authoritarian leadership roles. Researchers used the behavior of group members as their core data from which to make generalizations concerning leadership, decision making, group roles, and stages of group development.

Initially designed to be merely an experiential educational venture within the confines of an action laboratory, sensitivity training became more than that. The T-group process revealed a dormant need shared by many of the participants: an opportunity to talk about themselves and get honest reactions from others. Beyond the confines of the action laboratory, this behavior was considered immodest and impolite.

As a method of inquiry, sensitivity training made several methodological contributions to the search for integration. Before the advent of T-groups, social scientists had seen themselves as researchers and everyone else as actors or subjects. As a result of the action laboratory style of experiential inquiry, researchers and participants alike played both roles; and notions such as "trust building," "collaboration," "creative risk taking," and "feedback" became central concepts in the search for integration.

As sensitivity-training techniques matured, researchers generally agreed on what people could expect from a T-group experience: (1) self-insight, or some increase in self-knowledge, (2) an understanding of the forces that inhibit or facilitate group functioning, (3) an understanding of the interpersonal operations in groups, and (4) an opportunity to develop skills for diagnosing individual, group, and organizational behavior.[5]

The potential application of these processes to actual organizations was obvious. To introduce the lessons of the action laboratory into the decision-making and management levels of organizations, many social scientists began working as consultants with educational systems, industry, and volunteer associations. The researchers' rationale was that the action laboratory style of inquiry would enable individuals and organizations to become more aware of, and thereby exercise more control over, the process of integration. They expected that such awareness would enable the organization to become more productive and at the same time make the job a source of growth and human fulfillment for employees.

A number of organizations served as clients, and for a time, T-groups were a popular managerial innovation.[6] The results of these experiments are mixed, and it would be stretching the point to say that T-groups have made a substantial dent in the managerial philosophy of U. S. organizations. However, the T-group process did establish several important precedents for integration:

1. In addition to thinking and writing about organizations, social scientists for the first time actually dealt with them directly.

2. In investigating the nature of relationships among all levels of employees, some organizations began to experiment with changing behavior, attitudes, and social structures. Such experimentation had previously been reserved for product variables.

Some of the research carried out during this period deserves special mention as it put much of the investigation into individual/organization integration in a new light. The work of Douglas M. McGregor stands out.

The bridge builder: McGregor made two unique contributions to developing a method of inquiry for integration. First, he developed a very readable summary of what social scientists were discovering about the nature of man and explained how this discovery increases managers' options for accomplishing organizational objectives. Second, he made a standing invitation to managers themselves to engage in the process of experimentation and innovation.

It is curious that today McGregor is often seen more as an advocate for utopia than as a social scientist simply stating to managers that, under certain circumstances, individuals will actively seek responsibility, will exercise self-control, and will not inherently dislike work. He asserts that if managers accepted these assumptions about people (Theory Y) in place of the more accepted notions that derive from the sages (Theory X), their own role within the organization would have to change. Once he recognized that in most jobs the intellectual abilities of the average person are only partially used, the manager would have to learn how to create conditions that would allow members of the organization to achieve their own goals and at the same time direct their energies toward the success of the enterprise.

McGregor was very much a realist and acknowledged that perfect integration of employee needs with organizational objectives is not possible and that it remains management's prerogative to decide how and when to experiment. He suggested neither abdication nor permissiveness. The proposal to managers simply is, "If . . . we accept assumptions like those of Theory Y, we will be challenged to innovate, to discover new ways of organizing and directing human effort, even though we recognize that the perfect organization, like the perfect vacuum, is practically out of reach."[7]

The work of the early social scientists had focused on finding the proper form of inquiry. The applied social scientists tried to export the lessons they had learned in the action laboratories to organizations. (This is what the word *applied* in *applied social scientist* literally stands for.) In contrast, McGregor asked the manager to make and refine assumptions, to experiment, to test the results—in short, to see himself as a researcher and a learner. Indeed, McGregor's method of inquiry helped legitimize the manager as a researcher. (Unfortunately, the invitation to research has been lost in the debate over Theory X and Theory Y.) With McGregor, the social scientists' inquiry had reached into the heart of the matter.

THE PRACTITIONERS IN THE ORGANIZATION

As a result of McGregor's work, researchers saw the manager's style as a determining factor in the successful integration of individuals with the organization. Thus it became necessary for them to explore what goes into making a "good" manager and, if possible, to construct models of managers and their organizations at their peaks of effectiveness.

Using the scientific method: Robert R. Blake and Jane S. Mouton developed one of the more popular models used to describe managerial styles.[8] They plotted different patterns of leadership on a grid with two orthogonal axes calibrated from 1 to 9; one axis is labeled task needs and the other, individual needs. The grid exposes five "ideal" managerial styles: the slave driver (9,1), the country clubber (1,9) the compromiser (5,5), the invisible wonder (1,1), and the famous and most desirable managerial style (9,9) — the manager who can fully integrate the task and individual needs of his organization. Blake and Mouton also developed techniques and training programs to help the manager locate himself on their grid and develop ways to move toward the (9,9) style of integration.

Rensis Likert is another major empiricist who has searched for a stable set of parameters managers can use to judge the effectiveness and determine the style of their leadership. Concerned with the growing influence of individual consultants and the tendency clients have of selecting change strategies that are based on an individual practitioner's judgment or reputation, Likert wanted to establish a body of knowledge that would have greater empirical validity than the "shifting sands of practitioner judgment" generally do.

Toward this end Likert asked hundreds of managers across a wide variety of industries to describe the highest- and lowest-producing units in their organizations.[9] Using that information, he developed a series of continuum scales for decision making, motivation, leadership, goal setting, and organizational structure and divided each scale into four systems. System 1 describes traditional, authoritarian organizational behavior — one-man rule, discrete specialization, and the use of threat and fear as motivators. System 4, on the other hand, is characterized by collaborative decision making, interdependence, and intrinsic reward and motivational systems — an almost ideal integrative model.

Likert's research shows that when managers discuss their highest-producing units, they almost invariably describe System 3 or System 4 behavior, but that their descriptions of their lowest-producing units match System 1 behavior. He also shows that this pattern holds, irrespective of a manager's area.

Through different applications of the scientific method, social scientists arrived at similar conclusions about the potential for integration. Their conclusions might be thus summarized:

1. Integrating individual needs for affiliative ties and self-expression with an organization's need to produce is possible to a far greater degree than imagined before.

2. Organizations that have a high degree of integration are more productive than those that do not.

3. Rather than stifle an individual's growth and potential, organizations can contribute to them.

These findings were dramatically different from traditional beliefs that organizational and individual needs are incompatible; the shift in belief remains a source of confusion and disorientation. However, convinced of the validity of their findings and invited by corporation presidents, school superintendents, and hospital administrators, social scientists (now often called organizational development, or OD, practitioners) took their tools of inquiry into actual organizations. Their purpose was to alter the structures of organizations according to their data-based theories.

Changing and designing structures: Chris Argyris argues convincingly that managers have an enormous impact on their subordinates' growth and effectiveness or their lack thereof.[10] Nevertheless, he asserts that the typical structure of organizations and the behavior of their leadership often block employees' needs for self-direction and a sense of personal competence. The top managers' role is often that of the organization's gatekeepers who, through the use of power, rewards, and penalties, determine who gets ahead and who doesn't.

As a result of this authoritarianism, employees tend to be "leader centered"; at the expense of their own ideas and interests, they try to please the boss. Thus a boss/subordinate dependency relationship is created that hinders individuals from acquiring competence, defined by Argyris as the ability to solve problems and be in control of one's self and environment. The time-honored managerial principles—specialization of work, chain of command, unity of direction, and span of control—clearly enable managers to experience substantially more control of self and environment than their subordinates do.

The growing interest in organizational development as a promising avenue to integration has given rise to a number of idealized organizational models, many of which (like Likert's System 4) have their roots in Theory Y: organization renewal, organization revitalization, open systems, and temporary societies.[11]

Because there are a number of alternative models of organizational structure to choose from, dialogues between managers and OD practitioners tend to be carried on in either/or terms. Hence the "appropriate" organizational structure is oriented in either Theory X *or* Y; organizational structures should be permanent *or* temporary, or they should be hierarchical *or* open.

John J. Morse and Jay W. Lorsch have suggested, however, that because organizations are so different the issue of how to achieve integration cannot be resolved by determining which of the available models has the highest probability of motivating employees to achieve organizational objectives in a way that meets some of their own needs for competence.[12]

For instance, they describe a company with a highly formalized chain of command and elaborate, detailed policies for every conceivable situation, whose employees have minimal involvement in decisions—the classic authoritarian model; yet the employees are highly motivated and productive. They also know of a company where the structure is very flexible and employees have a large voice in decision making, but where people are neither motivated nor productive—a serious challenge to Theory Y! Both companies are manufacturing organizations where the majority of jobs are predictable, routine, and repetitive.

Nevertheless, two R&D companies that they examined show the reverse relationship between motivation/productivity and organizational structure. In one company, rigid policies and a formal chain of command reduced the motivation of researchers and scientists, while in the other, comparable organization conditions of greater individual autonomy heightened the scientists' motivation and productivity.

Morse and Lorsch conclude that there is no one best model of organizational structure. For them the appropriate structure depends on two factors:

1. The nature of the work. Repetitive, routine tasks might best be accomplished through the use of traditional principles of management, while the more abstract, conceptual work of scientists might best be accomplished under conditions of great individual autonomy.

2. The nature of the people. Morse and Lorsch agree with Argyris that all employees seek a sense of personal competence, and that they seek it in a complex variety of unique ways depending on how their need for a sense of competence interacts with the strengths of their other needs—for power, independence, structure, achievement, and affiliation.

In the companies they studied, Morse and Lorsch found that individual competence, motivation, and organizational productivity were more a function of the *fit* between task requirements, the particular competence needs of employees, and the organizational structure than a function of the particular organizational structure itself. More recent work has tended to confirm their findings.[13] The implication of these findings is that determining which design process fits an organization's structure is more conducive to integration than simply attempting to replace one structure with another.

Combining learning and doing: Members of the scientific profession rarely take an active role in applying new knowledge. Robert Oppenheimer, for instance, had little to say about the use of the atomic bomb. This is not so, however, for the social scientists pursuing the frontiers of individual and organizational integration; many are convinced that the methods used to discover and test emerging principles of integration can be employed by them in helping organizations achieve a greater degree of integration.

Calling themselves change agents (more recently, OD practitioners) and labeling their methods interventions, they introduced the scientific method, or at least a practical facsimile thereof, to the boardroom. To achieve their ends, they have to (1) collect data about the organization and the relationships among its members, (2) with the client form hypotheses based on these data as to what the underlying barriers to integration might be, (3) test and evaluate their hypotheses by using intervention methods such as T-groups, team building, and certain forms of job enrichment, and (4) make further statements and interventions as a result of their findings.

There seem to be three behavioral models that these change agents use in dealing with organizations:

1. By far the most popular model is that of the OD practitioner. This is the process design leader, the person who supplies methods for collecting valid data, feeds the data back, and plans and conducts interventions in collaboration with and in support of the manager-client. The OD practitioner is either a person external to the organization or a relatively low-power (staff rather than line) person inside. His conduct is guided by the general norms of scientific professionalism and democracy, and one of his main functions is to learn from and contribute to theory and technique building in the arena of planned organizational change. The practitioner's job is to help others solve their problems.

2. The second role model that change agents often employ is that of the Socratic consultant. Rather than lead and organize processes for inquiry, intervention, and change himself, the Socratic consultant views such activities as the responsibility of line management in an arena in which power is not only legitimate but also crucial. James A. Foltz, Jerry B. Harvey, and Jo Anne McLaughlin feel adamantly that "OD has to be a line activity. If it is not, it has no more impact on the functioning of an organization than a fundamentalist tent revival has on the operation of the Vatican."[14]

For the Socratic consultant, therefore, the essential conditions for OD to be successful are that it (1) respond directly to important organizational problems, (2) have a comprehensive theory that can be used for solving those problems, (3) be an extension of the chief executive officer, (4) enlist the power of all the managers in the organization, and (5) be supported by an OD staff that is competent in providing "Socratic consultation" assistance.

The consultant is clearly an aid to the change process under the direction of the CEO. Having made the initial decision to work with the company, the consultant makes few other substantive decisions. His role is to lay out the tools and resources of the behavioral sciences in menu form for the client and encourage him at least to taste exotic-looking dishes before deciding what to order. Like the practitioner, the consultant does not impose his values on the client; the purpose of the consultation is to support the CEO in his role as the manager of change.

3. The third role model, the advocate, is used by those who feel that social action, rather than any form of education or consultation, is called for if effective change is to occur. Advocates feel that although most forms of consultation and education (OD included) may advance the cause of integration, they can have no real impact on underlying cultural norms and social priorities. Instead of supporting the chief executive officer and helping him to facilitate change, the advocate/guerilla tries to make changes congruent with his own, not the client's, values.[15] The guerilla assumes change occurs only when power is diffused throughout the organization. Thus he works across and up and down the organization, seeking allies and building networks.

Far from collaborating with CEOs, the guerilla begins his change program by, for example, turning over evidence of organizational malfeasance to the media and other interested parties. He considers lawsuits, underground newspapers, and employee organizations as legitimate tools for change. He suffers no doubts about the appropriateness of imposing his agenda on the organization; such imposition is in fact his prime motivation. In place of the practitioner's hypothesis, the guerilla has a mission; in place of interventions, he has tactics; and in place of Socratic consultation, he marshals power and resources to serve his own objectives and values.

The three change-agent models I have discussed are currently used in organizations; however, there is, I feel, another resource managers could consider to achieve integration within their companies. Echoing the invitation issued by McGregor, I submit that creating an organizational climate that both encourages individual growth and ensures productivity can be a challenge and an opportunity for managers themselves.

THE MANAGER AS CHANGE AGENT: A ROLE REDEFINITION

Viewing their role from the perspective of organizational integration, managers could provide the leadership for designing the organization's structure to ensure a fit between task requirements and employee needs to feel competent. And this new role could incorporate and build on the manager's traditional activities: controlling, organizing, supervising, planning, and evaluating. These activities would still need to be performed, but they would be tailored to the particular needs of the organization's tasks and people. The basic processes for inquiry, design, and application have been developed and are ready for the manager to use.

The transition from the role of gatekeeper to change agent will be difficult. Once graduated from institutions of formal education, most people no longer find themselves rewarded for excellence in learning but instead are rewarded for excellence in meeting quarterly budgets, policy dictates, objectives, production quotas, and payrolls. A manager is rewarded for getting others to meet objectives for which he is responsible, not for facilitating individual development of competence. For many managers, the concept of themselves as the leader who integrates learning and doing within the organization is at odds with behavior that got them where they are. I would expect that managers may have some of the following concerns about seeing themselves as change agents:

"My employees would never be open with me." At first they may not be. Many things tend to confirm the suspicion that communication between levels in organizations is often distorted by fear and distrust: (1) the writings of theorists like Chris Argyris, (2) the OD practitioner's ethical standards of treating all comments as confidential, and (3) the awkward pause that usually follows after a CEO asks a first-line officer, "What do you think?"

Where mistrust and suspicion exist, they exist for a reason. The process of ferreting out that reason and responding to the data generated can not only build trust but also provide the manager with undistorted information to be used in designing a structure appropriate to his organization.

"I leave people problems to the psychologists." It does take some training to understand and work with personalities and individual behavior. However, managers generally have more people skills than they think they do. They use them in firing employees, deciding whom to promote, and in selecting someone to do a particular task. People problems are already part of a manager's job.

I do not mean to minimize the validity of these managers' sentiments, or of other reasons (for example, lack of time) they give for why they cannot assume an active leadership role in the area of organizational integration. The design of an organization's formal structure—its norms, policies, and rewards—is an activity traditionally delegated to personnel departments, training specialists, and OD practitioners.

I do mean to suggest that we need not continue to resign ourselves to a pyramidal organizational structure, which can in some cases make needs for individual competence incompatible with the organization's needs for productivity.[16] Further, I suggest that a current frontier in organizational life is active managerial leadership in the *process* of seeking organizational integration.

Where to begin: The manager himself can employ many methods of the practitioners with, I feel, multiple payoffs—methods for data collection (using interviews, questionnaires, and observation), for data feedback (summarizing the meat of the data and describing it to employees while engaging them in a discussion of what it means), for team building (developing a supportive climate in which employees can confront feelings and relationships), and for job enrichment (helping employees plan more effective and personally meaningful ways to get the job done). The manager would get to know his organization, employees would actually see their boss listen to and act on their concerns, and the modus operandi would be tailored to the unique needs of the organization.

Initially, a manager can expect resistance from both above and below to this role. To his superiors his actions may appear as an abdication of authority. And employees have been pretty well accustomed to not leveling with the boss except in crisis situations.

However, the aforementioned three roles that change agents assume offer a manager well-tested models that he could use to introduce integration within his own organization. Nevertheless, there are a number of pros and cons associated with the adoption of each of the models.

The advocate model, while a new and somewhat controversial role for OD practitioners, is not, I think, a strange concept to managers. Using power, building networks and alliances with selected people, developing tactics for programs and promotions, blowing the whistle (though this is usually done secretly to avoid recrimination), organizing employees around a pet idea, and giving information to newspapers, both above and below ground—these techniques are not new management practices. The board of directors that hires a new chief executive to "turn this place around" often seeks an advocate manager.

The major difference between the advocate and the other two models is that the advocate attempts to impose his personal conception of what the organization needs through dramatic alterations rather than by a gradual, developmental process. Also the advocacy style depends much more on the personal characteristics and abilities of the manager than on the use of learning methods and consultant skills. As such, the advocacy model entails the greatest personal risk and may well generate the most resistance, as well as energy and change.

The Socratic consultant's role, on the one hand, is lower keyed than that of the advocate and, on the other, less obtrusive than that of the traditional authority figure. The Socratic manager would act as a consultant to employees and work groups, who would make the final determinations. Of the three models, this one most requires that a manager relax his decision-making authority and accept the fact that his employees are responsible. Because of this, it may be the style least likely to be accepted by managers and employees. Thus, while I feel the Socratic role offers the greatest promise for organizational integration, it would be difficult for many executives to take this stance.

By contrast, the methods of the practitioner provide the manager with the information he needs to help the organization without placing him in a position that is either too active or too passive. Thus, of the three models, I see that of the practitioner as having the highest practical potential for success.

Even though the technology of change and learning has been developed to a remarkably sophisticated degree, we tend to separate learning from doing. Learning happens at places outside the organization or is invited in the person of an OD practitioner, while doing—getting the job done—is the order of the day at work. For managers, "getting the job done" will increasingly involve providing their employees with an enhanced sense of individual competence as well as with a paycheck. This will involve learning and doing for both managers and employees.

We live in an increasingly complex age in which an organization's survival and growth will depend on its ability to adapt and innovate rather than on its size and power. Assuming the leadership for organizational integration can help the manager create an organization flexible and strong enough to withstand the uncertainties ahead.

FOOTNOTES

1. For an incisive summary of the trends of the late eighteenth and nineteenth centuries, see Sheldon S. Wolin, *Politics and Vision: Continuity and Innovation in Western Political Thought.* Boston, Little, Brown & Co., 1960.

2. Roethlisberger, Fritz J., and Dickson, William J.: *Management and the Worker.* Cambridge, Harvard University Press, 1939.

3. Lewin, Kurt, Lippitt, Ronald, and White, Ralph K.: "Patterns of Aggressive Behavior in Experimentally Created 'Social Climates,'" *Journal of Social Psychology,* Vol. 10, 1939, p. 271.

4. See Leland P. Bradford, Jack R. Gibb, and Kenneth D. Benne, eds., *T-Group Theory and the Laboratory Method: Innovation in Re-Education.* New York, John Wiley & Sons, 1964.

5. Schein, Edgar H., and Bennis, Warren G.: *Personal and Organizational Change Through Group Methods.* New York, John Wiley & Sons, 1965.

6. See Chris Argyris, "T-Groups for Organizational Effectiveness," HBR March-April 1964, p. 60; Richard Beckhard, "Helping A Group with Planned Change: A Case Study," *Journal of Social Issues,* Vol. 15, No. 2, 1959, p. 13; and Sheldon A. Davis, "An Organic Problem-Solving Method of Organizational Change," *Journal of Applied Behavioral Science,* Vol. 3, No. 1, 1967, p. 3.

7. McGregor, Douglas M.: *The Human Side of Enterprise.* New York, McGraw-Hill, 1960, p. 54.

8. Blake, Robert R., and Mouton, Jane S.: *The Managerial Grid.* Houston, Gulf Publishing Company, 1964.

9. Likert, Rensis: *New Patterns of Management.* New York, McGraw-Hill, 1961.

10. Argyris, Chris: *Integrating the Individual and the Organization.* New York, John Wiley & Sons, 1964.

11. See Gordon L. Lippit, *Organizational Renewal: Achieving Viability in a Changing World.* New York, Appleton-Century-Crofts, 1969; Warren G. Bennis, *Organization Development: Its Nature, Origins, and Prospects.* Reading, Mass., Addison-Wesley Publishing Company, 1969; Eric L. Trist, "On Socio-Technical Systems" in Warren G. Bennis, Kenneth D. Benne, and Robert Chin, eds., *The Planning of Change,* 2nd ed. rev. New York, Holt, Rinehart & Winston, 1969, p. 272; Warren G. Bennis and Philip E. Slater, *The Temporary Society.* New York, Harper & Row, 1968; and Rensis Likert, *The Human Organization: Its Management and Value.* New York, McGraw-Hill, 1967.

12. Morse, John J., and Lorsch, Jay W.: "Beyond Theory Y," HBR May-June 1970, p. 61.

13. See Paul R. Lawrence, "Why the Change Worked," *Journal of Applied Behavioral Science,* Vol. 9, No. 5, 1973, p. 636; and Robert A. Luke, Jr., Peter Block, Jack M. Davey, and Vernon R. Averch, "A Structural Approach to Organizational Change," *Journal of Applied Behavioral Science,* Vol. 9, No. 5, 1973, p. 611.

14. Foltz, James A., Harvey, Jerry B., and McLaughlin, Jo Anne: "Organization Development, A Line Management Function," in John D. Adams, ed., *Theory and Method in Organization Development.* Arlington, Va., NTL Institute, 1974, p. 183.

15. Gregg, Roy G., and Van Maanen, John: "The Realities of Education as a Prescription for Organizational Change," *Public Administration Review,* November-December 1973, p. 522.

16. See Peter F. Drucker, "New Templates for Today's Organizations," HBR January-February 1974, p. 45.

INDEX

Page numbers in *italics* refer to illustrations; (t) indicates a table.